MACRO COOKBOOK

FOR BEGINNERS

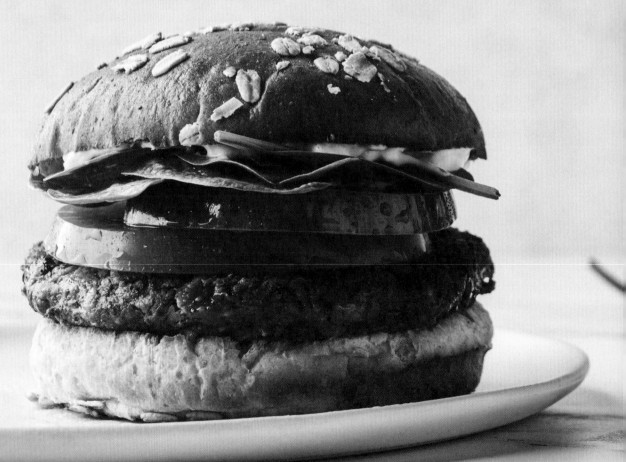

BLACK BEAN BURGER · PAGE 103

DEVIKA SHARMA, RD

PHOTOGRAPHY BY THOMAS J. STORY

MACRO
COOKBOOK
FOR BEGINNERS

Burn Fat and Get Lean
on the Macro Diet

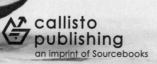

callisto
publishing
an imprint of Sourcebooks

Published by Callisto Publishing LLC C/O Sourcebooks LLC
P.O. Box 4410, Naperville, Illinois 60567-4410
(630) 961-3900
callistopublishing.com

Printed and Bound In China
OGP 17

*This book is
dedicated to everyone
who is ready to embrace
a new way of living.*

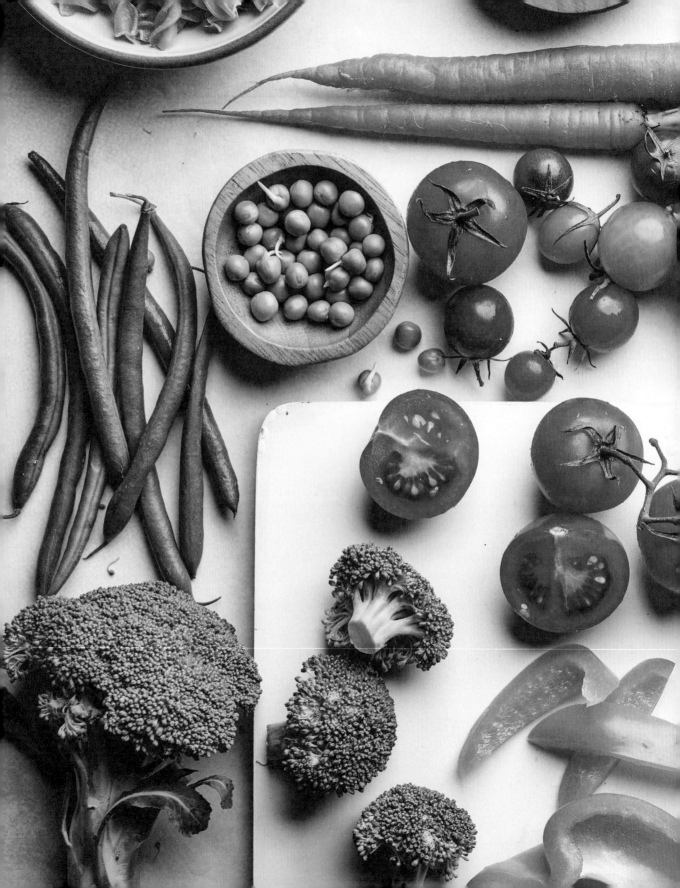

CONTENTS

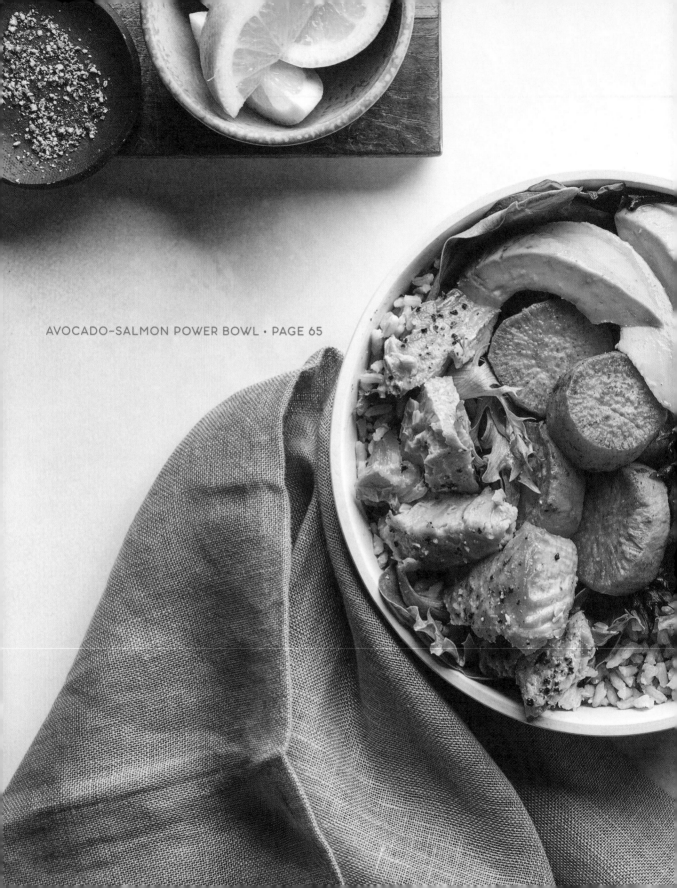

AVOCADO–SALMON POWER BOWL · PAGE 65

INTRODUCTION

If you're reading this book, it's likely because you've tried multiple diets but aren't seeing the results you want. Perhaps you continuously find yourself gaining and losing the same number of pounds, or maybe you're working out at the gym and not gaining muscle like you'd hoped. I get it—trust me, I do. Many diets promote a quick-fix approach that is rarely sustainable. The result? Frustration, disappointment, and possibly a negative relationship with food.

One can lose weight or get lean on any diet regardless of the quality of the food; however, for successful long-term results, food quality counts. That's where the macro diet comes in. Far from being another fad diet, it allows you to enjoy a full plate of protein, fat, and carbohydrates without feeling deprived.

I'm here to tell you that with patience, consistency, and the commonsense nutrition approach outlined in this book, you can achieve your health goals. As a registered dietitian, I have helped countless people reach their ideal weights and health goals. Although the journey for each person has been different, the end result has been the same: recognizing portion sizes for each macronutrient to best serve their body and goals.

My own weight loss journey taught me—and has allowed me to teach others—something important: Sustainable physical health comes with a shift in mindset. Switching your thinking from "I'm going on a diet" to "I'm changing the way I eat to fuel my body" will remove the feeling of restriction.

As the information, meal plan, and recipes in this book will show, you can fuel your body with nutritious and delicious foods and still achieve your health goals, whatever they may be.

CHOCOLATE-GRAHAM
CRACKER CUPS • PAGE 76

CHAPTER ONE

THE MACRO DIET EXPLAINED

It's time to say goodbye to all those diets that promise fast results but always leave you back at square one. Rather than missing out on the foods you love, say hello to a practical approach to eating that allows you to enjoy great food and achieve your health goals, be it to lose weight, build muscle, or get lean.

I've included my 14-day meal plan and 100 simple and satisfying recipes, but first I want to teach you about how macronutrients function in our bodies and why the macro diet promotes long-term health. Let's get started!

WHAT IS THE MACRO DIET?

In simple terms, the macro diet is a way of eating that focuses on tracking your daily macronutrient intake. Rather than avoiding certain foods, you use macros as a tool to find balance in your diet.

Three macronutrients make up every bite of food you eat: protein, carbohydrates, and fat. Although it's important to get the majority of your energy from nutrient-dense energy sources, no foods are off-limits on the macro diet as long as you stay within your daily macro targets. For this reason, it is sometimes referred to as the "if it fits your macros" (IIFYM) diet or "flexible eating." In other words, you can have your cake and eat it, too, as long as it fits your macros and the majority of your diet consists of high-fiber carbs, lean protein, and healthy fats.

Our bodies are often compared to cars that need fuel in the form of calories to function. And although this is true to some extent, it fails to take into account the *type* of fuel you put into your proverbial tank. Yes, you can derive energy from whatever calories you consume, but, behind the scenes, serious havoc may be unfolding. This, in turn, can impact your ability to manage your weight.

This book is going to show you how to calculate the correct quantity of macros and choose the best foods to support your daily macro targets.

WHY MANY DIETS FAIL

The big reason that so many modern diets fail is that they revolve around restriction, which, as many of us know, is hard to maintain in the long run. For instance, the low-carb keto diet means swearing off bread and pasta. When we focus on what we *can't* eat—rather than the foods we can and should fill our plate with—we encourage a cycle of craving, "slipups," and guilt that can promote an unhealthy relationship with eating.

Although it's true that you can shed pounds on crash diets when you expend more calories than you consume, this rapid weight loss often entails the loss of water and muscle, not just body fat. This is not desirable. Losing muscle mass impacts your metabolism because at rest, muscle burns more calories than fat.

All too often, these factors lead to weight cycling, which is the loss and gain of the same number of pounds before and after dieting. After depriving yourself of certain foods for a period of time, you are likely to feel more tempted than ever to eat them once a diet is finished. And rapid weight loss is often undone as you put back on water weight and have less muscle to help burn fat.

WHY THE MACRO DIET WORKS

The macro diet is not the new kid on the block. Rather than promising a new-found secret to get fit quick, it relies on tried-and-true principles of nutrition. We'll look in more detail at the science of the diet soon, but in simple terms, macro eating is so successful because it does away with the idea that you can never eat certain foods, because you can have them as long as you are hitting your daily macro targets.

As you'll learn, although no foods are off-limits, it's important to consume nutrient-dense foods most of the time to see results.

THE KEY HEALTH BENEFITS

The macro diet is adaptable to any lifestyle and schedule, and it offers many benefits for both the body and mind.

BETTER RELATIONSHIP WITH FOOD: The "all foods fit" approach allows you to enjoy your favorite foods without feeling deprived or guilty.

BUILDS MUSCLE: Although building muscle requires a combination of strength training and consuming more energy than you burn, adjusting your macro ratios—especially when it comes to protein—will help you build and preserve muscle tissue.

LONG-TERM HEALTH: Learning how to fuel your body with nutrient-dense meals like the recipes in this book—and eating less-healthy foods in moderation—can help you establish lifelong eating patterns that promote long-term health.

WEIGHT LOSS: Macro eating increases the awareness of food quality and quantity and allows better appetite control to support your weight goals. Consuming meals with adequate amounts of protein and healthy fats helps slow down the emptying of food from the stomach into the intestine. Consuming enough high-fiber carbohydrates adds bulk to food to slow down its passage through the body. Together, nutrient-dense sources of all three macronutrients will help you feel fuller.

RETHINKING YOUR ENERGY SOURCES

Before we look at how to adapt the macro diet to your needs in the next chapter, it's worthwhile to gain a better understanding of how macronutrients function in our bodies. Put simply, macronutrients are the three basic elements of food that your body requires in large amounts in order to function. Although some foods contain a combination of macros, most are skewed toward one or two.

Each macronutrient provides the body with energy (calories) in specific amounts. Although carbohydrates and protein provide 4 calories per gram, fats provide 9 calories per gram. During digestion, macronutrients are broken down into basic elements—protein into amino acid, carbs into sugar, and fat into fatty acids—which are absorbed by the bloodstream and then utilized by cells to produce energy.

The ratio of macronutrients you consume is expressed as a percentage of your total energy intake, so it will always add up to 100%.

What Macro Ratio Is the Best?

Although there is no one-size-fits-all approach to macros, as a starting point, this book focuses on a macronutrient ratio that is easy to achieve and allows for plenty of variety on your plate: 45% carbohydrates, 30% protein, and 25% fat. The meal plan in chapter 3 uses this as a weekly baseline ratio to help you lose weight.

In the long term, the best macro ratio is the one that best suits your body and lifestyle. For example:

→ Someone who is participating in endurance training will likely require more carbohydrates than a sedentary person, so their macronutrient ratio might look like this: 55% carbs, 25% protein, and 20% fat.

→ As a comparison, someone who is trying to build and maintain muscle mass may want to increase their protein intake so their macronutrient ratio might look like this: 45% carbs, 35% protein, and 20% fat.

Finding a macronutrient ratio that best suits your lifestyle and body may take some trial and error, but this chapter will equip you with the tools you need to calculate the ratio that meets your needs.

DO I STILL NEED TO COUNT CALORIES?

We already know that calories come from macros. By definition, when you are tracking your macros, you will always know exactly how many calories you have consumed in a day. What is important is that the total number of macros you consume correlates with the number of calories you require. You will need a deficit to lose weight and a surplus to gain muscle.

In this sense, it is important to recognize that not all calories are equal. For example, a chocolate bar and a handful of almonds may each have 200 calories, but the chocolate bar is going to be full of simple carbohydrates in the form of added sugar, which can cause your blood sugar level to spike, then quickly leave you feeling flat. What's more, it will lack the fiber, healthy fats, and proteins of almonds that keep you feeling full longer and provide sustained energy release.

Instead of approaching the macro diet as "giving up" calories, shift your mindset to focus on adding foods that will best help meet your carbohydrate, protein, and fat targets.

HAVE YOUR CAKE AND EAT IT, TOO

A good guideline to follow when it comes to how to balance wholesome foods and treats is the 80/20 rule. This means eating natural, wholesome foods like fresh produce most of the time (80%), leaving some room (20%) to enjoy treats or foods like cookies.

Here is a general rule to help maximize that 80% of your diet: divide your plate into three sections with half of the plate vegetables and fruits, a quarter of the plate lean protein, and a quarter of the plate whole grains and a source of healthy fat. With time, you'll be able to identify your macronutrient portions with ease, making this approach more sustainable.

A CLOSER LOOK AT MACROS

The diet industry bombards us with confusing and often conflicting messages around what we should and shouldn't eat. The truth is that no macronutrient is inherently "bad" for you, as long as you are eating enough of the right types. Although the recipes and meal plan in this book contain all the best sorts of macros to nourish your body, the following pages will teach you about the importance of each.

In Defense of Carbs

In recent decades, the success of the low-carb Atkins diet and more recently the ketogenic diet has made this macronutrient more maligned than any other. The truth of the matter is that eating carbs will not automatically cause you to gain weight; excess consumption of *any* macronutrient will.

Unlike protein and fat, carbs are the body's preferred energy source. They're broken down into sugar molecules (glucose) that cells readily take up and use as fuel. Although some glucose is stored as glycogen in muscles and the liver, excess may be converted into body fat.

Carbs are comprised of three components: fiber, starches, and sugars.

FIBER: Abundant in many foods like fruits and vegetables, fiber is unique in that it does not break down during digestion, which means that it has minimal caloric impact. Fiber helps with:

→ Bowel regulation and gut health
→ Improving blood cholesterol levels that support heart health
→ Controlling blood sugar levels

STARCHES: Made up of longer chains of sugar molecules, starches are referred to as complex carbs, which take longer to digest. This leads to less of a blood sugar spike, longer-lasting energy, and less hunger.

SUGARS: These are made up of one or a few sugar molecules, giving it the name "simple carbohydrates." Some sugars occur naturally (like in fruit) and others are added into foods (like table sugar). According to the 2015– 2020 Dietary Guidelines for Americans and Heart and Stroke Canada, added sugars should be limited to less than 10% of total daily calories. Unlike naturally occurring sugars that are found in foods that contribute other nutrients and fiber, added sugars provide no nutritional value.

> **TAKEAWAY MESSAGE:** *Although you should limit your intake of added sugars, you should consume a variety of wholesome carbs that provide long-lasting energy, keep you feeling full longer, and deliver essential nutrients to your body. Good sources of carbs are listed on pages 22–23 in chapter 2.*

The Power of Protein

There is a good reason protein has celebrity status when it comes to weight loss: it requires more energy to digest than other macronutrients. In other words, it has a greater thermic effect, one of the components that impacts metabolism.

Protein provides energy and is part of every cell in the body. Proteins are made up of multiple building blocks known as amino acids, some of which the body synthesizes on its own (nonessential) and others that need to be obtained from the diet (essential).

Essential amino acids must be consumed daily because they cannot be stored in the body, and limited amounts impact the production of muscle and body tissue proteins. By consuming a diet that includes a variety of protein sources, one can obtain adequate amounts of essential amino acids.

Protein is best known for its role in the growth and repair of body and muscle cells, in particular with exercise. Consuming adequate amounts of protein after a workout provides the body with the amino acids it needs to decrease muscle breakdown and support muscle growth—muscle burns more calories than fat at rest. Other functions of protein include:

→ Producing enzymes, hormones, and body chemicals to carry out metabolic reactions

→ Transporting nutrients

→ Muscle contraction

→ Promoting the feeling of fullness

TAKEAWAY MESSAGE: *Protein helps us build muscle and burn fat. Consume various protein sources daily to nourish your body with amino acids, the building blocks of our cells. See page 23 in chapter 2 for good sources of protein.*

Why You Need Fats

Despite what you may have heard, fats are an essential nutrient that your body needs. Although it's true that low-fat diets were once the "it" thing to lose weight, research actually suggests that this information is outdated, and for good reason. Fats are a part of every single cell in your body, making it impossible to live without them. Some of the main functions of fats include:

→ Absorbing and transporting fat-soluble vitamins (A, D, E, K)

→ Slowing down the emptying of food from the stomach into the intestine, which promotes the feeling of fullness

→ Producing hormones

→ Regulating cholesterol levels and heart health

It's important to note that not all dietary fats (saturated, trans, polyunsaturated, monounsaturated) are created equally nor are they automatically stored as body fat. In fact, weight gain and an increase in body fat occurs when any nutrient is consumed more than the body requires. Since the type of dietary fat impacts the body differently, it's important to choose wisely.

Solid fats (trans and saturated) can raise low-density lipoprotein (LDL), known as "bad" cholesterol, which is linked to higher risk of cardiovascular disease. On the contrary, unsaturated fats (monounsaturated and polyunsaturated) can help improve the levels of high-density lipoprotein (HDL), known as "good" cholesterol.

THE SUPPORTING CAST: MICRONUTRIENTS

There is one final category of nutrients that we haven't looked at yet: micronutrients. Although they are only needed in small amounts and are not a source of energy, they provide essential vitamins and minerals that allow your body to function at an optimal level.

They also play a huge role in metabolic reactions, including energy metabolism, which involves a series of biochemical reactions that enzymes support. Some of these enzymes require coenzymes or cofactors, of which many are vitamins. For example, thiamine (vitamin B_1) is involved in carbohydrate metabolism. A deficiency in thiamine could not only impact this process but can manifest as neurological disorders.

How do you make sure you are consuming enough micronutrients? A good approach is to "eat the rainbow"—that is, consume a variety of different-colored fruits and vegetables.

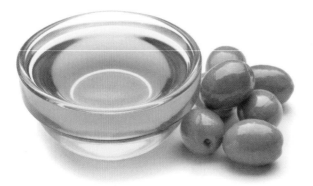

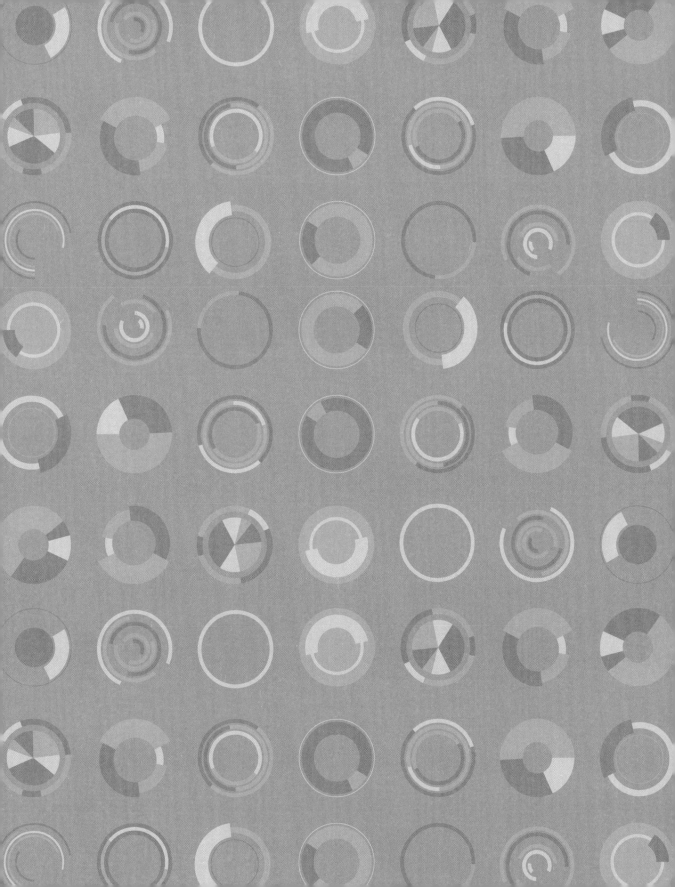

GREEK CHICKPEA
POWER BOWL · PAGE 58

MAKING THE MACRO DIET WORK FOR YOU

This chapter teaches you how to calculate how many macros you should be consuming each day for your body and fitness goals. This will provide a clear path to achieve those goals and establish long-term healthy eating patterns.

The meal plan in chapter 3 is designed as a starting point for weight loss, giving you structure around what to eat during the course of two weeks. It can be easily adapted, whether your goal is to maintain your current weight or build muscle.

THE 5 STEPS TO MACRO SUCCESS

There are five key steps to help you find success with the macro diet: decide your goal, calculate your daily calories, calculate your daily macros, plan for success, and track your daily numbers.

Step 1: Decide Your Goal

Creating a specific, measurable, achievable, relevant, and time-framed (SMART) goal will help keep you focused. For example, if your goal is "to lose weight," that's not specific enough. A better approach to this would be: "In three months, I want to be 8 pounds lighter. I will track my macros to ensure I'm meeting my protein-energy requirements, weigh myself monthly, and use the fitting of my jeans to monitor my progress."

LOSING WEIGHT

The meal plan in chapter 3 is designed to result in at least 1 pound of weight loss per week. With that said, there is some nuance to weight loss that is important to understand.

You probably have heard of the "3,500-calorie rule." That is, to lose 1 pound of fat in a week, one must burn 500 calories or eat 500 calories less every day for the week (3,500 calories total). With this approach, one technically should lose around 20 pounds in 5 months, right? Unfortunately, that's not necessarily the case. It doesn't take into account that our bodies differ in metabolic rate and genetics. So, although this approach may work in the short term, it's important to recognize that weight loss is not straightforward or linear, and adjustments will need to be made to your overall intake.

There are no hard-and-fast rules around exercising to lose weight while tracking your macros; however, healthy eating combined with consistent physical activity does support a more sustainable lifestyle change. To maintain a healthy body weight, build strength, and reduce your risk of disease, the Canadian Physical Activity Guidelines recommend healthy adults 18 to 64 get a minimum of 150 minutes of moderate to vigorous aerobic activity weekly and muscle-bone strengthening activities twice weekly. Examples of moderate intensity physical activity include brisk walking and bike riding. Examples of vigorous activity would be jogging and cross-country skiing. Muscle-strengthening activities include push-ups, sit-ups, lifting weights, and climbing stairs.

GAINING LEAN MUSCLE

The macro diet is also a popular way of eating to build muscle. This is because it gives you control over how much energy you are consuming each day—especially when it comes to energy from protein—so that you can consume a surplus of calories required to add weight and grow muscle.

MAINTAINING GOOD HEALTH

The macro diet is not just for weight loss or gain—it's also ideal for maintaining your health in the long run.

Step 2: Calculate Your Daily Calories

Now that you've decided on your goal, let's figure out how many calories you need. You can calculate this manually using the following calculations or use an online calculator like NIDDK.NIH.gov/bwp. The benefit of calculating manually is that you gain a deeper understanding of how factors such as age and physical activity impact your overall energy needs.

FIND OUT HOW MUCH ENERGY YOU USE AT REST: You first need to know your basal metabolic rate (BMR), which is the number of calories your body uses at rest each day to sustain basic functioning.

To begin, you need to know what your height and weight are in metric units. Divide your weight in pounds by 2.2 and round it up or down to the nearest whole figure to find out the kilograms. Then multiply your height in inches (1 foot = 12 inches) by 2.54 and round it up or down to calculate the centimeters. Make note of these figures. Next, fill out the calculation for your sex below, taking into account your weight, height, and age:

BMR MALE: (10 × WEIGHT IN KG) + (6.25 × HEIGHT IN CM) – (5 × AGE) + 5 = ...

BMR FEMALE: (10 × WEIGHT IN KG) + (6.25 × HEIGHT IN CM) – (5 × AGE) – 161 = ...

FIND OUT HOW MUCH ADDITIONAL ENERGY YOU USE: The next step is to determine how much additional energy you burn through physical activity each day by choosing an activity factor as follows:

→   1.2 if you are sedentary (little to no exercise)
→   1.375 if you are lightly active (light exercise or sports 1 to 3 days per week)
→   1.55 if you are moderately active (moderate exercise or sports 3 to 5 days per week)
→   1.725 if you are very active (hard exercise or sports 6 to 7 days per week)
→   1.9 if you are extremely active (hard and/or heavy daily exercise or sports)

Once you know your BMR and activity factor, you can calculate your total daily energy expenditure (TDEE) by multiplying the numbers together:

So, your BRM x your activity factor (from above) = your TDEE _____

This number is a fairly accurate measurement of the average total energy your body burns every day.

To make more sense of the above numbers, let's see how they add up for a real person. For example, Jane is a 30-year-old moderately active woman who weighs 165 pounds and is 5 foot 4 inches tall, which equals 64 inches. Dividing her weight in pounds by 2.2, she writes down that she is 75 kilograms. Multiplying her height in inches by 2.54, she notes that she is 163 centimeters tall.

She can figure out her BMR using the formula for women:

$$(10 \times 75) + (6.25 \times 163) - (5 \times 30) - 161 =$$
$$750 \quad + \quad 1{,}019 \quad - \quad 150 \quad - 161 = \underline{\textbf{1,458 CALORIES}}$$

(HER BMR – THE MINIMUM AMOUNT OF ENERGY HER BODY NEEDS)

TDEE = BMR X MODERATELY ACTIVE FACTOR
$$= 1{,}458 \times 1.55 = \underline{\textbf{2,260 CALORIES}}$$

(THE DAILY AMOUNT OF ENERGY SHE NEEDS TO MAINTAIN HER WEIGHT)

ADJUST CALORIES IF YOU WANT TO LOSE WEIGHT

As a guideline, you can subtract 250 to 500 calories from your TDEE to find out how many calories you need to consume per day to lose weight.

TDEE – 500 CALORIES = CALORIES TO CONSUME EACH DAY FOR WEIGHT LOSS

For Jane, this would be 2,260 – 500 = 1,760 calories.

I really do believe caloric intake should not be less than 1,400 calories per day. Anything lower makes it difficult to consume essential nutrients, and as a comparison, 1,200 calories is what a sedentary seven-year-old child should be consuming. The goal is *healthy* weight loss with a flexible eating pattern. Instead of over-restriction, consume enough nutrient-dense foods and adjust your lifestyle to burn more calories.

ADJUST CALORIES IF YOU WANT TO GAIN MUSCLE

To gain muscle, add 250 to 500 calories to your TDEE. This should be done in conjunction with strength training exercise. The sources of calories matter here, too, so make sure to fuel your body with, high-fiber carbohydrates, healthy fats, and lean proteins, such as those listed on pages 22–24.

Step 3: Calculate Your Daily Macros

Now that you know how many calories you need to lose weight, it's easy to figure out how many grams of each macronutrient you need to eat daily. The calculations are not absolute. It's a framework built around an average weekly macronutrient ratio that provides adequate intakes of essential nutrients; you may decide you prefer a different macro intake because of your needs or tastes. This is fine, so long as you consume enough food to satisfy what are known as the acceptable macronutrient distribution ranges (AMDR). Per the 2015–2020 Dietary Guidelines for Americans, AMDR for people's daily intake of calories are 45% to 65% carbohydrates, 10% to 35% protein, and 20% to 35% fat. Eating within these ranges is vital to support tissue growth, facilitate energy production, and prevent disease related to nutritional deficiency. The meal plan in this book uses the average weekly macro ratio of 45% carbohydrates, 30% protein, and 25% fat for both weight loss and weight maintenance. Using an average ratio accommodates the 80/20 rule, which allows you to eat a varied diet.

IF YOU WANT TO LOSE OR MAINTAIN WEIGHT

Let's start with calculating the grams of macros to consume each day if you are wanting to lose weight. Remember:

- → Carbohydrates provide 4 calories per gram and will make up 45% of total daily calories
- → Protein provides 4 calories per gram and will make up 30% of total daily calories
- → Fat provides 9 calories per gram and will make up 25% of total daily calories

Let's calculate Jane's macros. She needs 1,760 calories per day for weight loss.

JANE'S NEEDS

MACRONUTRIENT	MACRONUTRIENT RATIO		DAILY CALORIE NEEDS		CALORIES PER MACRONUTRIENT		CALORIES PER GRAM		DAILY MACRONUTRIENT GRAMS
CARBOHYDRATES	0.45	×	1760	=	792	÷	4	=	198
PROTEIN	0.30	×	1760	=	528	÷	4	=	132
FAT	0.25	×	1760	=	440	÷	9	=	49

JANE'S DAILY WEIGHT LOSS NEEDS ARE:

1,760 CALORIES   198G CARBS   132G PROTEIN   49G FAT

YOUR NEEDS

MACRONUTRIENT	MACRONUTRIENT RATIO		DAILY CALORIE NEEDS		CALORIES PER MACRONUTRIENT		CALORIES PER GRAM		DAILY MACRONUTRIENT GRAMS
CARBOHYDRATES	0.45	×	_____	=	_____	÷	4	=	_____
PROTEIN	0.30	×	_____	=	_____	÷	4	=	_____
FAT	0.25	×	_____	=	_____	÷	9	=	_____

YOUR DAILY WEIGHT LOSS NEEDS ARE:

_____ CALORIES   _____G CARBS   _____G PROTEIN   _____G FAT

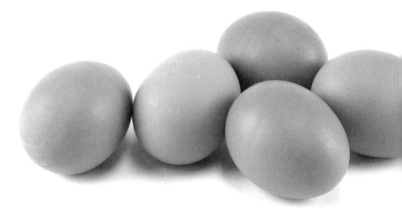

IF YOU WANT TO BUILD MUSCLE

To build muscle, you can do the same calculations as above, but add 250 to 500 calories to your TDEE (rather than subtracting) and increase the ratio of protein you consume in order to promote muscle growth. A good starting point for this is 45% carbs, 35% protein, 20% fat.

HOW PRECISELY DO I NEED TO HIT MY DAILY TARGETS?

Eating exactly the right number of grams of any given macronutrient per day is easier said than done. For this reason, it's okay to leave some wiggle room from day to day, as long as across the week they average out close to your daily macro target and macro ratio.

Although there is no hard rule as to how much you can be outside of your macro ratio split, I recommend you do not consume more or less than 5% of a particular macro in your ratio split. If you continuously are above or below this range, it's a good indication that you need to adjust your targeted macronutrient ratio to meet this need.

Step 4: Plan for Success

It's often said that failing to plan is planning to fail. Given the importance of hitting your daily macro targets to achieve results, you will need to plan your nutrition ahead of time.

To get you started, the 14-day meal plan in chapter 3 provides an easy entry to the diet, with shopping lists to make the nutritious recipes from this book.

Beyond the first 14 days, you should plan your weekly eating schedule. Think about what an average day looks like to you and write down how many meals you eat. Next, attempt to evenly split your macros across each meal. If your goal is 120 grams of protein per day, and you eat three meals, you'd want to aim for 40 grams for each meal. This groundwork makes hitting your macros much more manageable rather than trying to get all of one type of macro in one sitting. Once you have a general split, you can scale macro allotments up or down for different times of day.

Once you have this, it is important to plan your shopping, food prep, and cooking to save time putting together meals to avoid scrambling to find the right foods at the last minute. Here are some useful tips to help you throughout the week:

→ Set aside some time every week to plan your meals and create a grocery list.
→ Check to see what foods you have on hand before doing your shopping.
→ Batch cook for multiple days so that you have meals already prepared.
→ Find meals that you love to eat that fit your macro profile and cook those frequently.

Step 5: Track Your Daily Numbers

For any new skill, you need to practice before you become good at it. Understanding and tracking macros is no different. If you don't know what or how much to eat, you may feel so overwhelmed that you feel like throwing in the towel by eating whatever is in front of you. Remember, although it may seem detail-oriented at first, this is a short-term approach until you have a better understanding of the macro content of different foods. Eventually, it'll become second nature and you won't need to track.

It's okay if your macro intake is out of range some days due to hunger levels. There are many factors that can impact hunger (e.g., hormones). Acknowledge your hunger cues by eating something nutrient-dense that will promote fullness (e.g., protein + fiber). There may be days where you overeat because of other reasons (e.g., boredom). Identify and address the root cause. When it happens (because it will happen), just keep moving forward. Go easy on yourself—you're only human. Do not compensate by eating less the next day or skipping meals—you still need the energy and nutrients to function well.

Here are some apps that can make tracking easier: MyFitnessPal, Macros-Calorie Counter, and MyPlate Calorie Tracker. Although each one offers a different way to log food consumed, they provide insight into how much food you've consumed daily and the amount of each macronutrient. When you plan your meals ahead of time, you can enter them into the app and adjust your intake accordingly. Alternatively, you can track your own macros using an Excel spreadsheet and looking up the nutritional information for each food using a reputable nutrient database like USDA Food Data Central (ndb.nal.usda.gov/index.html).

THE BEST FOODS TO EAT

Now that you have your framework for macro eating, it's time to fill it in with your favorite foods. This is where you can get creative and have some fun. Of course, the 14-day meal plan in chapter 3 does the planning for you, but if you are creating a new weekly menu or adjusting it for your fitness goals, the recipes in this book include nutritional calculations so you know exactly how many macros are in each serving.

When following the macro diet, you could technically eat processed foods all day and in theory still lose weight, if that is your goal. Although you can do that, you really need to ask yourself if you should.

Processed foods require the body to use less work to break them down. For example, consuming orange juice doesn't require much processing, and it is passed from the stomach to the intestine rather quickly. If you were to consume the whole orange, though, digestion would take longer, starting from the chewing.

This does not mean you can't enjoy foods that are more processed. You absolutely can, but as you read on page 6, they should only make up 20% of your diet. What happens if you overindulge one night? Breathe and move on. Calories are not the be-all and end-all, and the weight loss journey is never linear.

The recipes in this book are designed to maximize nutrition without sacrificing flavor, so you'll see that it will contain foods (like maple syrup) that are often shunned by fad diets. Luckily, this is not another fad diet. Let's look at some of the ingredients you can enjoy to maximize nutrition.

Foods with Healthy Carbs

There are many different sources of carbohydrates, so it's important to include a variety in your diet. The goal is to limit added sugars and consume more nutrient-dense and high-fiber carbohydrates like vegetables and whole grains. Many carbohydrate foods contain a mix of simple and complex carbs. Here are some highly nutritious sources of carbohydrates:

SIMPLE CARBOHYDRATES

→ apples

→ bananas

→ berries

→ milk

→ oranges

→ yogurt

COMPLEX CARBOHYDRATES

→ beans
→ lentils
→ peas

→ potatoes
→ quinoa
→ rice

→ rolled oats
→ whole-grain or
whole wheat bread

Foods with Healthy Fats

It is important to consume quality unsaturated fats (monounsaturated, polyunsaturated) and limit your intake of saturated fats. Below are ten different sources of healthy fats you should be including in your diet. You'll find most of them in the recipes and meal plans provided.

→ avocados
→ olive oil
→ nuts (e.g., almonds,
walnuts)

→ nut butter (e.g.,
100% all-natural
peanut butter)
→ olives

→ seafood (e.g., fish)
→ seeds (e.g., sun-
flower, pumpkin)

Foods with Quality Proteins

One of the best approaches to consuming enough protein is to include a source with each meal along with eating a variety of protein sources. Here are some examples of protein sources:

ANIMAL-BASED PROTEIN

→ Boneless, skinless
chicken breast
→ Eggs

→ Extra-lean ground
beef
→ Seafood

→ Tuna, canned
in water

PLANT PROTEIN

→ Beans
→ Hummus

→ Lentils
→ Nuts (e.g., peanuts)

→ Soy nuts, soybeans
→ Tofu and tempeh

→ Low-fat cheese (e.g., cheddar, cottage)

→ Low-fat milk

→ Soy milk

→ Yogurt (e.g., plain Greek yogurt)

ARE SUPPLEMENTS OKAY?

Certain supplements can be beneficial for some people, but they cannot replace food. Food offers much more than just macronutrients. It provides us with micronutrients, phytonutrients, fiber, and—importantly—pleasure.

If you're considering a protein supplement to meet your macro target, hold that thought. Although this may be warranted for some health conditions, like for healing after surgery, most healthy adults can meet their protein requirements from meals and snacks.

When it comes to micronutrients, you should also prioritize food before pills. Of course, there may be some people who require supplementation of a particular nutrient—such as folic acid to support pregnancy or iron for anemia—but there may be some situations where a supplement can interact with drugs. Before reaching for a pill, talk to your doctor.

Supplements are often marketed as beneficial, but not all of them have enough scientific background to support the claims. It's not uncommon for supplements to be full of filler ingredients whose safety and effectiveness remains unclear.

HYDRATION, REST, AND RELAXATION

Achieving good health can take patience and consistency, but it should include self-care. After all, we are only as good as our bodies will let us be. It's important to take time to relax, reduce stress, and ensure you are logging an adequate amount of sleep.

HYDRATION: A key player that sometimes is overlooked is hydration. Our fluid needs differ daily since there are many factors (e.g., physical activity, sex) that can influence it. Water should always be your go-to choice for hydration. It's an essential nutrient that has zero calories or sugar. If you don't consume enough fluids, dehydration can occur, bringing with it headaches, digestive problems, and dizziness. This won't support your well-being and can present a different set of challenges to reaching your fitness goals. Typically, adult women require 9 cups of fluid per day, while adult men require 12 cups.

REST: Sleep times vary according to age-group, and it is recommended that adults get 7 to 9 hours a day. Sleep impacts our appetite, which may impact our food choices. Levels of appetite-regulating hormones, ghrelin (hunger hormone) and leptin (fullness hormone), vary with sleep. Sleep deprivation can cause ghrelin to increase and leptin to decrease, resulting in increased hunger levels and the potential to consume more food than needed. This can lead to increased body fat.

RELAXATION AND STRESS REDUCTION: Self-care goes beyond eating well, good hydration, and enough sleep. Engaging in positive self-talk and activities that support relaxation can help increase body awareness, reduce stress, impact mood, and diminish negative self-judgments, factors that can often present as challenges when trying to lose weight. Dedicate at least 30 minutes of your day to yourself to engage in a non-food-related activity that makes self-wellness a priority. Some common activities include home yoga, meditation, a walk outside, or writing in a gratitude journal.

Above all, remember that macro eating is not a fad diet about restricting your food consumption to get fast results. It's about finding a nutrient balance to support your fitness objectives and making informed food choices to sustain long-term health.

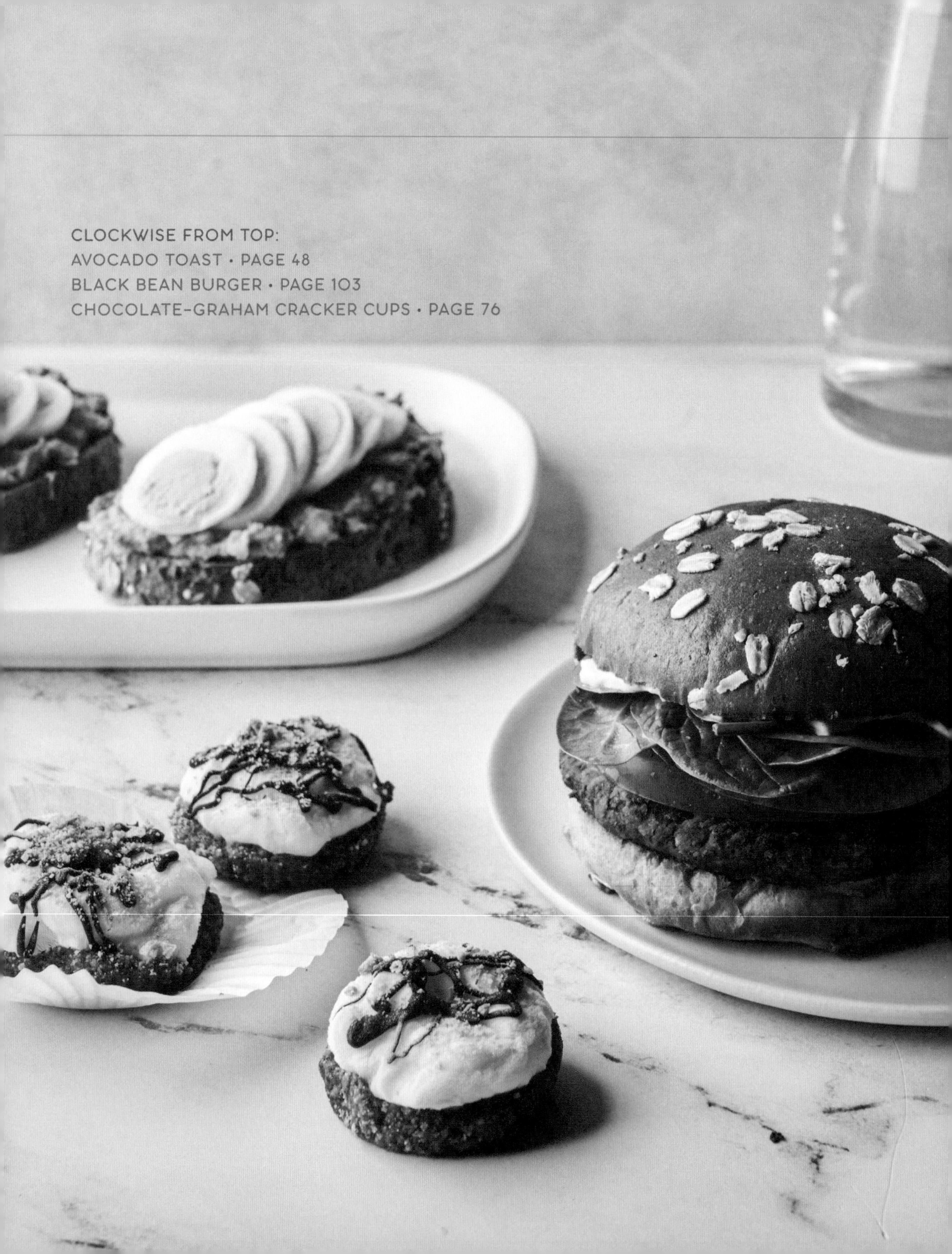

CLOCKWISE FROM TOP:
AVOCADO TOAST • PAGE 48
BLACK BEAN BURGER • PAGE 103
CHOCOLATE-GRAHAM CRACKER CUPS • PAGE 76

CHAPTER THREE

THE 14-DAY MEAL PLAN

Getting fit and healthy can seem daunting—especially on diets that require you to give up your favorite foods or eat bland ones. Cue the 14-day meal plan that is going to show you that achieving your weight goals should not be restrictive or stressful, but fun. Think about all of the foods you can eat and add to your diet instead of stressing out about the ones you can't. Why? All foods fit when tracking macronutrients.

ABOUT THE MEAL PLAN

The meal plan is designed as an introduction to losing weight with macro eating. It reflects the macro ratio guidelines from the previous chapter, which is a weekly average ratio of 45% carbohydrates, 30% protein, and 25% fat. Using an average ratio allows for more meal variety and less restriction and supports the 80/20 lifestyle. The daily caloric intake will vary, though the plan has been designed for an average sedentary person to lose 1 to 2 pounds per week. Remember, slow and steady wins the race, and weight loss is not linear.

The menu is designed for two people but can be halved if you're eating solo. To help save time and cost, meals have been created so that leftovers can be consumed the next day.

Tailoring the Meal Plan to Your Needs

You may decide to follow the meal plan as-is to familiarize yourself with macro eating and see what results you achieve in 14 days. However, if you wish to have it meet the macro needs you calculated in the previous chapter, you can scale the meals up or down to match your targets.

For example, if you are a man with greater macro needs than this plan is designed for, you could increase the meal serving sizes by 25%. Or, if you are trying to build muscle, you can increase your overall macro targets and increase your protein ratio, following the macro guidelines on page 18 and adding more sources of protein to your diet with foods such as those on page 23.

Become familiar with foods that are easily scalable and enjoyable to eat. For example, adding more rice would increase your carbohydrate intake, adding more chicken would impact protein intake, and adding more olive oil would increase your fat intake. Many of the recipes in the book give examples of how you can adjust the meal to better meet your macronutrient ratio. To find out yourself how many macros certain foods contain, you can use a website like USDA Food Data Central (ndb.nal.usda.gov/index.html) or apps such as My Fitness Pal (see Resources on page 154). Regardless of how you adjust the macronutrients, be sure that they convert to meet your daily calorie target. Energy balance is the driving force behind weight loss or muscle gain.

Snacks and Desserts

Snacks are a good way to sneak in nutrition to help meet your macronutrient ratio. When chosen wisely, they can help ward off hunger pangs. When trying to decide on a snack that will keep you feeling full, consider pairing a protein and high-fiber food source together (e.g., nonfat Greek yogurt with berries). As mentioned in chapter 2, unlike many fad diets, tracking macros provides flexibility with food choices, including desserts. The meal plan includes portion-controlled treats to show you how an 80/20 approach to eating can help meet weight goals while still enjoying the foods you eat. Remember, all foods fit when tracking your macros.

Now, let's get cooking!

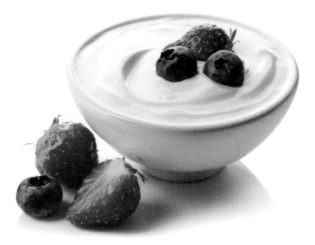

MEAL PLAN: WEEK 1

	BREAKFAST	LUNCH	DINNER	DESSERT/SNACK
MONDAY	PB & J Overnight Oats (page 41)	Cucumber-Chicken Wraps (page 114)	Shrimp, Peanut, and Rice Bowl (page 67)	–
TUESDAY	Avocado Toast (page 48)	*Leftover:* Shrimp, Peanut, and Rice Bowl (page 67)	Beef Spaghetti (page 137)	Chewy Banana Bites (page 75) crumbled over ½ cup plain nonfat Greek yogurt
WEDNESDAY	*Leftover:* PB & J Overnight Oats (page 41)	*Leftover:* Beef Spaghetti (page 137)	Cashew Chicken Bowl (page 61)	Chewy Banana Bites (page 75)
THURSDAY	*Leftover:* Avocado Toast (page 48)	*Leftover:* Cashew Chicken Bowl (page 61)	Black Bean and Mushroom Quesadillas (page 104)	Chewy Banana Bites (page 75) crumbled over ½ cup plain nonfat Greek yogurt
FRIDAY	*Leftover:* PB & J Overnight Oats (page 41)	*Leftover:* Black Bean and Mushroom Quesadillas (page 104)	Garlic-Chicken Burger (page 113)	Chewy Banana Bites (page 75)
SATURDAY	Go Green Smoothie (page 39)	*Leftover:* Garlic-Chicken Burger (page 113)	Baked Salmon with Green Beans (page 122)	½ cup low-fat vanilla ice cream with 1 cup raspberries
SUNDAY	Cheesy Chive and Egg Sandwich (page 50)	Maple-Ginger Chicken Stir Fry (page 115)	*Leftover:* Baked Salmon with Green Beans (page 122)	½ cup low-fat vanilla ice cream with ¾ cup fresh raspberries

WEEK 1 MEAL PLAN GROCERY LIST

Dairy & Alternatives

- [ ] Cheddar cheese, low-fat shredded (¾ cup)
- [ ] Feta cheese, low-fat crumbled (½ cup)
- [ ] Greek yogurt, nonfat plain, 2 (750g) containers
- [ ] Milk, skim (1½ cups)
- [ ] Mozzarella cheese, reduced-fat shredded (½ cup)
- [ ] Parmesan cheese, reduced-fat shredded (¼ cup)
- [ ] Vanilla ice cream, low-fat (2 cups)

Meat & Alternatives

- [ ] Beef (1 pound)
- [ ] Black beans (15 ounces)
- [ ] Chicken (48 ounces)
- [ ] Egg whites, 1 (500ml) carton
- [ ] Eggs, large (5)
- [ ] Salmon (16 ounces)

Grains

- [ ] Bread, 100% whole-grain or whole wheat (6 slices)
- [ ] Brown rice
- [ ] Buns, 100% whole-grain (4 each)
- [ ] Oats, rolled
- [ ] Spaghetti, whole-grain
- [ ] Tortilla, 100% whole wheat (6 [10-inch] tortillas)

Nuts & Alternatives

- [ ] Almond butter, all-natural (2 tablespoons)
- [ ] Almonds, whole (¼ cup)
- [ ] Cashews, unsalted (2 tablespoons)
- [ ] Chia seeds (6 tablespoons)
- [ ] Flaxseed, ground (2 tablespoons)
- [ ] Hemp hearts (4 tablespoons)
- [ ] Peanut butter, 100% all-natural creamy (⅔ cup)
- [ ] 70% dark chocolate chips (1.25 ounces)

Pantry Items

- ☐ Balsamic vinegar
- ☐ Black pepper
- ☐ Cayenne pepper
- ☐ Chili powder
- ☐ Cooking spray, nonstick
- ☐ Dried oregano
- ☐ Garlic powder
- ☐ Ground cinnamon
- ☐ Ground cumin
- ☐ Italian seasoning
- ☐ Lemon juice
- ☐ Lime juice
- ☐ Low-sodium soy sauce
- ☐ Maple syrup
- ☐ Olive oil
- ☐ Sea salt
- ☐ Sriracha
- ☐ Vanilla extract
- ☐ Worcestershire sauce

Produce

- ☐ Avocado, large (1)
- ☐ Bananas, large (3)
- ☐ Bell pepper, green (1)
- ☐ Blueberries (6 ounces)
- ☐ Carrots, large (5)
- ☐ Cilantro (1 bunch)
- ☐ Crushed tomatoes, 1 (28-ounce) can
- ☐ Cucumber, large (1)
- ☐ Garlic bulbs (3)
- ☐ Ginger (1)
- ☐ Green beans (4 cups)
- ☐ Mixed greens (4 cups)
- ☐ Raspberries (30 ounces)
- ☐ Scallions (13)
- ☐ Shallot (1)
- ☐ Spinach, baby (9 cups)
- ☐ Tomato, large (2)
- ☐ White button mushrooms, whole (4 cups)
- ☐ White onion, medium (1)
- ☐ Yellow pepper, large (1)

MEAL PLAN: WEEK 2

	BREAKFAST	LUNCH	DINNER	DESSERT/SNACK
MONDAY	Greek Yogurt Parfait (page 40)	Black Bean and Corn Chicken Salad (page 56)	Sweet Crispy Tofu Bowl (page 100)	–
TUESDAY	Mushroom-Feta Egg Cups (page 49)	*Leftover:* Sweet Crispy Tofu Bowl (page 100)	Chicken Parmesan (page 118)	Chocolate–Graham Cracker Cups (page 76)
WEDNESDAY	*Leftover:* Greek Yogurt Parfait (page 40)	*Leftover:* Chicken Parmesan (page 118)	Teriyaki Beef and Broccoli Bowl (page 64)	–
THURSDAY	*Leftover:* Mushroom-Feta Egg Cups (page 49)	*Leftover:* Teriyaki Beef and Broccoli Bowl (page 64)	Spicy Chicken and Rice Bowl (page 63)	Chocolate–Graham Cracker Cups (page 76) with an apple
FRIDAY	*Leftover:* Greek Yogurt Parfait (page 40)	*Leftover:* Spicy Chicken and Rice Bowl (page 63)	Black Bean Burger (page 103)	Chocolate–Graham Cracker Cups (page 76)
SATURDAY	Blueberry Cheesecake Oatmeal and Egg White Scramble (page 47)	*Leftover:* Black Bean Burger (page 103)	Pineapple-Shrimp Bowl (page 120)	1 cup nonfat Greek yogurt with ½ cup fresh raspberries
SUNDAY	PB & Banana French Toast (page 46)	Turkey Meatballs and Zoodles (page 112)	*Leftover:* Pineapple-Shrimp Bowl (page 120)	½ cup low-fat vanilla ice cream with ½ cup fresh raspberries

> Double-check your pantry items before going grocery shopping; some foods were purchased in week 1.

Dairy & Alternatives

- ☐ Cheddar cheese, low-fat shredded (⅔ cup)
- ☐ Egg whites, 2 (500ml) cartons
- ☐ Eggs, large (8)
- ☐ Feta, low-fat crumbled (¾ cup)
- ☐ Greek yogurt, nonfat plain (7 cups)
- ☐ Milk, skim (1 cup)
- ☐ Mozzarella, reduced-fat shredded (¼ cup)
- ☐ Parmesan, reduced-fat shredded (⅔ cup)
- ☐ Ricotta cheese, low-fat (¼ cup)

Meat & Alternatives

- ☐ Beef, extra-lean (1 pound)
- ☐ Black beans, canned, 2 (15-ounce) cans
- ☐ Chicken, boneless, skinless breasts (3 pounds)
- ☐ Shrimp (1 pound)
- ☐ Tofu, extra-firm (14 ounces)
- ☐ Turkey, extra-lean ground (9 ounces)

Nuts & Seeds

- ☐ Almonds, slivered (⅓ cup)
- ☐ Flaxseed, ground (2 tablespoons)
- ☐ Hemp hearts (3 tablespoons)
- ☐ Peanut butter, 100% all-natural creamy (6 tablespoons)
- ☐ Pepitas (4½ tablespoons)
- ☐ 70% dark chocolate chips (0.5 ounce)

Pantry Items

- [ ] All-purpose flour
- [ ] Chili powder
- [ ] Cinnamon
- [ ] Cooking spray, olive oil
- [ ] Cornstarch
- [ ] Fajita seasoning
- [ ] Freshly ground black pepper
- [ ] Garlic powder
- [ ] Graham cracker, crumbles
- [ ] Honey
- [ ] Italian Seasoning
- [ ] Ketchup
- [ ] Lime juice
- [ ] Maple syrup
- [ ] Marinara sauce (2 cups)
- [ ] Oregano, dried
- [ ] Paprika, smoked
- [ ] Pesto sauce
- [ ] Raisins, dried (½ cup)
- [ ] Soy sauce, reduced sodium
- [ ] Sriracha
- [ ] Vanilla extract

Produce

- [ ] Apples, red small (2)
- [ ] Banana (1)
- [ ] Bell pepper, red large (2)
- [ ] Blueberries (½ cup)
- [ ] Broccoli (2 cups)
- [ ] Carrots, medium (2)
- [ ] Cherry tomatoes (2 cups)
- [ ] Cilantro, fresh
- [ ] Corn kernels, frozen (½ cup)
- [ ] Cucumber, small (1)
- [ ] Dates, dried, pitted (½ cup)
- [ ] Edamame, frozen, shelled (3 cups)
- [ ] Garlic bulbs (4)
- [ ] Mango chunks (1 cup)
- [ ] Mixed greens (12 cups)
- [ ] Mushrooms (2 cups)
- [ ] Pineapples (½ cup)
- [ ] Raspberries (4 cups)
- [ ] Scallions (8)
- [ ] Spinach, baby (1 cup)
- [ ] Tomato, large (1)
- [ ] White onion, small (1)
- [ ] Zucchini, medium (3)

Whole Grains

- [ ] Bread, 100% whole-grain (12 slices)
- [ ] Bread crumbs
- [ ] Brown rice
- [ ] Buns, 100% whole wheat (4)
- [ ] Oats, rolled (2½ cups)
- [ ] Puffed rice cereal (½ cup)
- [ ] Quinoa

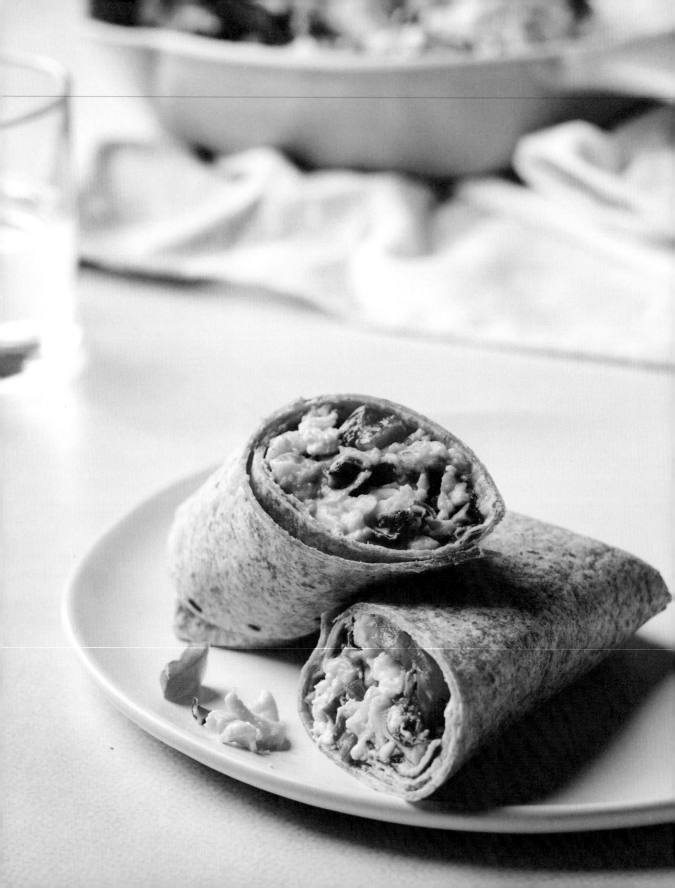

CHAPTER FOUR

BREAKFASTS

PEANUT BUTTER–BANANA SHAKE

If you like peanut butter sandwiches, then you'll love this shake. To help with satiety, it contains a source of protein (Greek yogurt) and fiber (oats) in addition to the carbs (bananas) and healthy fat (peanut butter). The recipe is easily scaled down by dividing all of the ingredients by 4.

4 small bananas

2 cups 1% milk

1¼ cups rolled oats

1 cup nonfat plain
   Greek yogurt

4 tablespoons creamy
   100% all-natural
   peanut butter

1 ounce dark chocolate
   (optional)

1. Combine the bananas, milk, oats, Greek yogurt, peanut butter, and chocolate (if using) into a blender and puree until smooth.

2. Pour into 4 glasses and serve.

3. Refrigerate any leftovers in a mason jar for up to 24 hours. Shake well before serving.

> **SUBSTITUTION TIP:** Not a fan of peanut butter? Use almond butter, which will leave you feeling just as satisfied.

PER SERVING: Calories: 449; Fat: 15g; Total Carbohydrates: 61g; Net Carbs: 53g; Fiber: 8g; Protein: 22g; Sodium: 80mg

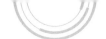

GO GREEN SMOOTHIE

When in doubt, smoothie it out—especially if you're short on time. Smoothies are a great way to fuel your body, as long as they include foods that promote fullness. Smoothies tend to empty out of the stomach faster than solid foods, so it's important to include a source of protein, a healthy fat, and a high-fiber carbohydrate.

3 cups fresh baby spinach

1 large banana

1 cup skim milk

1 cup nonfat plain
  Greek yogurt

½ cup fresh blueberries

⅓ cup rolled oats

⅛ cup 100% all-natural
  almond butter

1 tablespoon hemp hearts

1. Combine the spinach, banana, milk, yogurt, blueberries, oats, almond butter, and hemp hearts in a blender and puree until smooth.

2. Pour into 2 glasses and serve.

> **LEFTOVER TIP:** Refrigerate leftovers in a mason jar for up to 24 hours. Shake well before serving.

PER SERVING: Calories: 383; Fat: 11g; Total Carbohydrates: 49g; Net Carbs: 42g; Fiber: 7g; Protein: 26g; Sodium: 135mg

GREEK YOGURT PARFAIT

Serves 6 · Prep time: 5 minutes / Cook time: 10 minutes
30 MINUTES OR LESS, VEGETARIAN

It's important to consume protein with each meal, and Greek yogurt is a great source of it. Three quarters of a cup of Greek yogurt provides about 15 grams of protein. There are many different ways to enjoy Greek yogurt, and this meal is another example of how you can easily start your day off with protein, healthy fats, and fiber.

2¼ cups rolled oats

¾ cup slivered almonds

6 tablespoons puffed
  rice cereal

6 tablespoons raisins

4½ tablespoons
  hemp hearts

4½ tablespoons pepitas

¾ teaspoon ground
  cinnamon

6 cups nonfat plain
  Greek yogurt

4½ cups fresh raspberries

1. Cook the oats in a nonstick skillet over medium heat, stirring continuously, until lightly brown, 2 to 3 minutes. Transfer the browned oats to a large bowl.

2. Add the almonds, rice cereal, raisins, hemp hearts, pepitas, and cinnamon to the oats and mix well. Divide the mixture into 6 servings.

3. To assemble the parfaits: Layer each of 6 glasses with ½ cup of Greek yogurt, ¼ cup of raspberries, a ¼ serving of the oat mixture, ½ cup of Greek yogurt, ¼ cup of raspberries, and the remaining ¼ serving of the oat mixture. Serve immediately.

LEFTOVER TIP: Store the yogurt, oat mixture, and berries separately and assemble on the day you plan to eat it to maximize flavor.

PER SERVING: Calories: 460; Fat: 14g; Total Carbohydrates: 52g; Net Carbs: 43g; Fiber: 9g; Protein: 35g; Sodium: 96mg

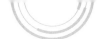

PB & J OVERNIGHT OATS

Serves 6 · Prep time: 10 minutes / Cook time: 8 hours or overnight
VEGETARIAN

This is one of the easiest breakfasts to prepare, and the best part is that you can assemble several jars at one time and have them ready for the week. Looking to change up the Greek yogurt? Substitute with a soy-based yogurt fortified with vitamin D and calcium.

6 cups nonfat plain
  Greek yogurt
3 cups rolled oats
6 tablespoons chia seeds
4½ cups fresh raspberries
6 tablespoons creamy
  100% all-natural
  peanut butter

1. Combine 1 cup of the Greek yogurt, ½ cup rolled oats, and 1 tablespoon of chia seeds in each of 6 mason jars and mix well.

2. Cover and refrigerate overnight to let the oats absorb the liquid.

3. To serve, add ¾ cup of berries and 1 tablespoon of peanut butter to each mason jar and enjoy.

> **SUBSTITUTION TIP:** The peanut butter can be replaced with 2 tablespoons of almond butter.

PER SERVING: Calories: 515; Fat: 17g; Total Carbohydrates: 56g; Net Carbs: 40g; Fiber: 16g; Protein: 40g; Sodium: 99mg

CINNAMON-RAISIN BAGELS

Makes 6 bagels · Prep time: 15 minutes / Cook time: 25 minutes
NUT-FREE, VEGETARIAN

Many commercially prepared bagels are much larger and have extra calories and carbohydrates. The great thing about making your own bagels is that you can manipulate the size to help fit your carbohydrate intake.

Nonstick cooking spray

¾ cup all-purpose flour, plus more for dusting

¼ cup oat flour

2 teaspoons baking powder

1 teaspoon ground cinnamon

½ teaspoon sea salt

⅛ teaspoon ground nutmeg

⅓ cup raisins

1 cup nonfat plain Greek yogurt

1 teaspoon vanilla extract

1 large egg, beaten

1. Preheat the oven to 375° F. Lightly grease a donut pan and set aside.

2. In a medium bowl, mix the all-purpose flour, oat flour, baking powder, cinnamon, salt, nutmeg, and raisins.

3. Add the yogurt and vanilla and mix with a fork until crumbly and well combined.

4. Lightly dust a work surface with flour. Knead the dough, being careful not to overwork it, about 8 times.

5. Divide the dough into 6 pieces. Roll each piece into a 6- to 7-inch rope. Place each dough rope in the donut pan and pinch the ends together to form a complete circle. Brush the dough with the beaten egg.

6. Bake for 20 to 25 minutes, or until lightly browned. Let the bagels cool completely on a wire rack.

7. Store the bagels in an airtight container in the refrigerator for up to 3 days.

> **PREP TIP:** If you don't have a donut pan, line a baking sheet with parchment paper and pinch the ends of the dough together to securely seal it.

PER SERVING (1 BAGEL): Calories: 115; Fat: 1g; Total Carbohydrates: 18g; Net Carbs: 17g; Fiber: 1g; Protein: 8g; Sodium: 130mg

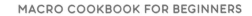

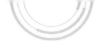

BLUEBERRY–LEMON AND CHIA MUFFINS

Makes 12 muffins · Prep time: 15 minutes / Cook time: 25 minutes
NUT–FREE, VEGETARIAN

Chia seeds are loaded with healthy fats, fiber, and minerals. They are great with pudding, sprinkled on top of a salad, or in muffins—like these.

Nonstick cooking spray

2 cups all-purpose flour

2 tablespoons chia seeds

1 tablespoon lemon zest,
   plus ½ tablespoon
   for garnish

1 teaspoon baking soda

1 teaspoon baking powder

¼ teaspoon sea salt

1 cup nonfat plain
   Greek yogurt

½ cup, plus 1 tablespoon
   maple syrup

¼ cup olive oil

1 tablespoon 1% milk

1 large egg, whisked

1 tablespoon freshly
   squeezed lemon juice

1 cup fresh blueberries

1. Preheat the oven to 375° F. Line a 12-cup muffin tin with liners. Lightly spray the liners with nonstick cooking spray.

2. In a large bowl, mix the flour, chia seeds, lemon zest, baking soda, baking powder, and salt. Set aside.

3. In a medium bowl, mix the yogurt, maple syrup, olive oil, milk, egg, and lemon juice.

4. Pour the wet ingredients into the dry ingredients and carefully stir until just mixed. Do not overmix. The batter will be thick. If it is too thick, mix in an additional 1 tablespoon of milk.

5. Add the blueberries and gently fold them into the batter with a rubber spatula. Divide the batter equally into the prepared muffin cups, and garnish with remaining lemon zest.

6. Bake for 20 to 22 minutes, or until baked through. Transfer the muffin tin to a wire rack and let cool for 5 minutes before removing the muffins from the pan and cooling completely.

> **PREP TIP:** Test the muffins for doneness with a toothpick. If it comes out clean, the muffins are cooked. If not, continue to bake for a few more minutes.

PER SERVING (1 MUFFIN): Calories: 193; Fat: 6g; Total Carbohydrates: 30g; Net Carbs: 28g; Fiber: 2g; Protein: 5g; Sodium: 161mg

VANILLA–STRAWBERRY PROTEIN PANCAKES

Serves 3 · Prep time: 1O minutes / Cook time: 2O minutes
NUT-FREE, 3O MINUTES OR LESS

If you feel like having pancakes with extra nutritional value, give these a try. The Greek yogurt and milk provide protein, while the chia seeds and strawberries provide some fiber. If you're looking to increase protein, pair the pancakes with scrambled eggs, turkey bacon, or tofu bacon.

1 cup all-purpose flour

1 tablespoon chia seeds

½ teaspoon
baking powder

½ teaspoon baking soda

1 large egg, beaten

¾ cup nonfat plain
Greek yogurt

⅓ cup 1% milk

2 tablespoons
maple syrup

1 teaspoon vanilla extract

1 cup diced strawberries

Nonstick cooking spray

1. In a large bowl, mix the flour, chia seeds, baking powder, and baking soda.

2. In another bowl, mix the egg, yogurt, milk, maple syrup, and vanilla. Add the wet ingredients to the dry ingredients and mix well. Add the strawberries and carefully fold them into the batter with a rubber spatula. Let the batter sit for 5 minutes.

3. Lightly spray a large skillet with nonstick cooking spray. Pour ¼ cup of batter into the pan and cook until golden brown, 2 to 3 minutes on each side. Repeat with the remaining batter to make a total of 6 pancakes. Serve immediately

> **SUBSTITUTION TIP:** Not a fan of strawberries? Replace them with fresh blueberries and still get a punch of flavor and fiber.

PER SERVING (3 PANCAKES): Calories: 306; Fat: 4g; Total Carbohydrates: 52g; Net Carbs: 48g; Fiber: 4g; Protein: 15g; Sodium: 273g

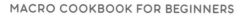

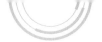

PEANUT BUTTER AND CHOCOLATE WAFFLES

Serves 4 · Prep time: 15 minutes / Cook time: 10 minutes
30 MINUTES OR LESS, VEGETARIAN

Waffles seem to be a very popular food these days. There are so many ways to enjoy them: chicken and waffles, waffle sticks, and even waffle grilled cheese sandwiches. Here is an easy way to enjoy them and pack in some protein.

2 cups all-purpose flour

2 tablespoons unsweetened cocoa powder

1½ tablespoons baking powder

¼ teaspoon sea salt

1¼ cups 1% milk

⅔ cup nonfat plain Greek yogurt, plus more as desired

2 large eggs, whisked

1 teaspoon vanilla extract

2 tablespoons dark chocolate chips

Nonstick cooking spray

4 tablespoons creamy 100% all-natural peanut butter

1. Preheat the waffle maker according to the manufacturer's instructions.

2. In a large bowl, mix the flour, cocoa powder, baking powder, and salt.

3. In another bowl, mix the milk, Greek yogurt, eggs, and vanilla. Pour the wet ingredients into the dry ingredients. Add the chocolate chips and carefully stir until just combined. Do not overmix.

4. Lightly spray the hot waffle maker with nonstick cooking spray. Pour ½ cup of batter into the center of the waffle maker and cook according to the manufacturer's instructions. Repeat with the remaining batter. Cut each waffle into 4 sections. Place 6 sections on each plate, spread 1 tablespoon of peanut butter on each serving, and top with extra Greek yogurt, as desired.

> **INGREDIENT TIP:** To increase the peanut butter flavor, replace ⅓ of the all-purpose flour with powdered peanut butter. It also increases the protein content.

PER SERVING (6 WAFFLE SECTIONS): Calories: 432; Fat: 13g; Total Carbohydrates: 60g; Net Carbs: 54g; Fiber: 4g; Protein: 21g; Sodium: 265g

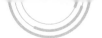

PB & BANANA FRENCH TOAST

Serves 2 · Prep time: 10 minutes / Cook time: 10 minutes
30 MINUTES OR LESS, VEGETARIAN

This version of French toast increases the amount of protein by using eggs, peanut butter, and Greek yogurt. It also reduces the need for added sugars like maple syrup since it is sweetened by the natural sugars from the banana. As a means to maximize the protein, scramble any remaining egg mixture and serve it alongside the French toast.

2 large eggs

½ teaspoon plus
⅛ teaspoon ground
cinnamon, divided

¼ teaspoon vanilla extract

2 tablespoons creamy
100% all-natural peanut
butter, divided

4 slices 100%
whole-grain bread

1 small banana, cut
into slices

Nonstick cooking spray

1 cup nonfat plain
Greek yogurt

1. In a shallow bowl, beat together the eggs, ½ teaspoon of cinnamon, and vanilla. Set aside.

2. Spread 1 tablespoon peanut butter on 1 slice of bread, top with half of the banana slices, and close with the second slice of bread to make a sandwich. Repeat with the remaining 2 slices of bread.

3. Lightly spray a skillet with nonstick cooking spray and set over medium heat.

4. Carefully soak both sides of the sandwich in the egg mixture. Cook the sandwich in a skillet until golden brown, 2 to 4 minutes on each side. Repeat with the remaining sandwich.

5. Sprinkle the sandwiches with the remaining ⅛ teaspoon cinnamon and serve with the Greek yogurt.

> **COOKING TIP:** If any of the egg mixture remains, spray the skillet with additional nonstick cooking spray, add the remaining egg mixture, and cook the eggs, stirring with a wooden spoon until scrambled. Serve on the side with the sandwiches. This will ensure that you meet your protein intake for this meal.

PER SERVING: Calories: 430; Fat: 16g; Total Carbohydrates: 42g; Net Carbs: 35g; Fiber: 7g; Protein: 31g; Sodium: 373mg

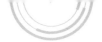

BLUEBERRY CHEESECAKE OATMEAL AND EGG WHITE SCRAMBLE

Serves 2 · Prep time: 5 minutes / Cook time: 10 minutes
30 MINUTES OR LESS, VEGETARIAN

Serving oatmeal is a great way to add fiber to your breakfast. It's also easy to flavor it with spices like cinnamon, fruits like berries, and nut butters. I've added ricotta cheese, which makes the oatmeal slightly thicker, and the addition of the graham crackers provides a touch of sweetness and texture like a cheesecake crust. The blueberries have natural sugars, making it feel like you're eating dessert for breakfast.

1 cup skim milk

⅛ teaspoon sea salt, plus more for seasoning

½ cup rolled oats

4 tablespoons low-fat ricotta cheese

½ cup fresh blueberries

⅛ cup almonds

2 teaspoons crushed graham crackers

1 teaspoon olive oil

1¼ cups egg whites

½ cup shredded low-fat cheddar cheese

Freshly ground black pepper

1. In a medium saucepan over medium-high heat, bring the milk and ⅛ teaspoon of salt to a boil. Add the oats, lower the heat to medium, and cook, stirring occasionally, until tender, 5 to 6 minutes. Remove from the heat, cover, and let sit for 2 to 3 minutes.

2. Add the ricotta cheese to the oat mixture and stir to combine. Add the blueberries and gently stir. Top with the almonds and crushed graham crackers.

3. In a medium skillet, heat the olive oil over medium heat. Add the egg whites and cook without stirring until the edges begin to set. Using a wooden spoon, gently stir the eggs, forming large curds, until cooked through. Turn off the heat, add the cheese, and season with salt and pepper. Spoon the oatmeal into bowls and serve the eggs on a plate on the side.

> **SUBSTITUTION TIP:** To make this meal gluten-free, use gluten-free oats and omit the graham crackers.

PER SERVING: Calories: 373; Fat: 13g; Total Carbohydrates: 29g; Net Carbs: 25g; Fiber: 4g; Protein: 36g; Sodium: 700mg

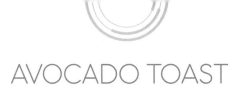

AVOCADO TOAST

Serves 4 · Prep time: 5 minutes / Cook time: 15 minutes
NUT-FREE, 30 MINUTES OR LESS, VEGETARIAN

Avocado toast has made its mark in the breakfast category, and for good reason. The healthy fat from the avocado, combined with the protein from the eggs and fiber from whole-grain toast, will help promote fullness.

4 large eggs

1 avocado, pitted
and peeled

1 cup crumbled low-fat
feta cheese

2 teaspoon cay-
enne pepper

1 teaspoon freshly ground
black pepper

½ teaspoon sea salt

2 teaspoons freshly
squeezed lemon juice

8 slices 100% whole-grain
bread, toasted

1. Put the eggs in a small saucepan, add water to cover by 1 inch, and bring to a boil over high heat. Cover with a lid, turn off the stove, and let the eggs sit for 12 minutes. Discard the water and run the eggs under cold water.

2. While the eggs are cooking, in a large bowl, mash the avocado with a fork.

3. Add the feta, cayenne pepper, black pepper, salt, and lemon juice and mix well.

4. Top each slice of toast with ¼ of the avocado and feta mixture. Serve with the hard-boiled eggs.

> **COOKING TIP:** To add more flavor without changing the nutrient profile, increase the cayenne pepper, salt, and pepper to taste.

PER SERVING (2 SLICES AVOCADO TOAST AND 1 HARD-BOILED EGG):
Calories: 330; Fat: 17g; Total Carbohydrates: 30g; Net Carbs: 22g;
Fiber: 8g; Protein: 16g; Sodium: 593g

MUSHROOM–FETA EGG CUPS

Serves 4 · Prep time: 10 minutes / Cook time: 20 minutes

30 MINUTES OR LESS, VEGETARIAN

Although eggs are a great source of protein, hard-boiled eggs are not everyone's cup of tea. These egg cups are a great way to add flavor and increase your vegetable intake at breakfast.

Nonstick cooking spray

2 cups halved cherry
   tomatoes

2 cups chopped white
   button mushrooms

6 scallions, green parts
   only, chopped

½ cup crumbled low-fat
   feta cheese

8 large egg whites,
   plus 4 whole large
   eggs, beaten

Sea salt

Freshly ground
   black pepper

2 tablespoons creamy
   100% all-natural
   peanut butter

8 slices 100% whole-grain
   bread, lightly toasted

1. Preheat the oven to 350° F. Lightly spray 12-cup muffin tin with nonstick cooking spray.

2. Divide the tomatoes, mushrooms, and scallions equally in the 12 muffin cups. Top each with the feta. Pour the egg whites equally over the vegetables. Season with salt and pepper.

3. Bake for 20 minutes, or until the egg is set. Remove the egg cups from the muffin tin and place 3 on each of 4 plates. Spread the peanut butter equally on the slices of toast and place 2 on each plate. Serve immediately.

> **LEFTOVER TIP:** Refrigerate any leftover egg cups in an airtight container for up to 4 days. Reheat the cups for about 30 seconds in the microwave oven before serving.

PER SERVING: Calories: 299; Fat: 11g; Total Carbohydrates: 31g; Net Carbs: 25g; Fiber: 6g; Protein: 21g; Sodium: 517mg

CHEESY CHIVE AND EGG SANDWICH

Serves 2 · Prep time: 10 minutes / Cook time: 10 minutes
NUT-FREE, 30 MINUTES OR LESS, VEGETARIAN

If you're looking for a way to add more protein to a meal without changing the fat-macronutrient ratio, consider adding egg whites, which are loaded with protein. If you're looking to add more volume to the meal, load them up with vegetables like mushrooms, tomatoes, bell peppers, and spinach. This will also add more fiber and a variety of nutrients.

1¼ cups egg whites

1 tablespoon dried chives

¼ teaspoon sea salt

½ tablespoon olive oil

⅛ cup shredded low-fat cheddar cheese

2 slices 100% whole-grain bread, lightly toasted

1 cup fresh baby spinach, thinly sliced

2 thick tomato slices

1. In a small bowl, beat the egg whites. Add the chives and salt and mix well.

2. In a medium skillet, heat the oil over medium heat. Add the egg whites and cook without stirring until the edges begin to set. Using a wooden spoon, gently stir the eggs, forming large curds, and cook until the eggs are set, 2 to 3 minutes. Remove from the heat.

3. Add the cheese and stir, letting the cheese melt. Place 1 slice of toast on each of 2 plates. Divide the egg mixture equally onto the toast and top with the spinach and tomato slices. Serve immediately.

> **LEFTOVER TIP:** If there are any leftovers, store the egg mixture, toast, spinach, and tomatoes in separate airtight containers and assemble just before serving.

PER SERVING: Calories: 210; Fat: 6g; Total Carbohydrates: 14g; Net Carbs: 11g; Fiber: 3g; Protein: 23g; Sodium: 654mg

GOAT CHEESE AND TOMATO BREAKFAST WRAP

Serves 4 · Prep time: 5 minutes / Cook time: 15 minutes
NUT-FREE, 30 MINUTES OR LESS, VEGETARIAN

Vegetables for breakfast? Yes! Every meal is an opportunity to sneak them in, especially when combined with the right ingredients. You can easily add more vegetables like mushrooms to these wraps to help increase the volume of the meal.

4 large eggs

⅓ cup 1% milk

¼ teaspoon freshly ground black pepper

¼ teaspoon sea salt

1 tablespoon olive oil

4 cups fresh baby spinach

¼ cup crumbled goat cheese

2 scallions, green parts only, finely chopped

4 large 100% whole wheat tortillas

1 Roma tomato, diced

1. In a medium bowl, whisk together the eggs, milk, pepper, and salt. Set aside.

2. In a large skillet, heat the olive oil over medium heat. Using a basting brush, evenly coat the pan with the oil. Add the spinach and cook until it starts to wilt, about 1 minute.

3. Pour the eggs into the skillet and cook until the eggs begin to set, about 2 minutes. Using a wooden spoon, gently stir the eggs, forming large curds, and cook until the eggs are set, 2 to 3 minutes. Remove from the heat, add the goat cheese and scallions, and stir to combine.

4. To assemble the wraps: Spoon equal amounts of scrambled egg into the middle of each of 4 tortillas. Top with the diced tomatoes. Fold in the sides of the tortillas and roll into a wrap.

COOKING TIP: Feel free to warm up the tortillas on a dry skillet for 30 seconds prior to filling them with scrambled egg mixture.

PER SERVING: Calories: 270; Fat: 14g; Total Carbohydrates: 23g; Net Carbs: 18g; Fiber: 5g; Protein: 14g; Sodium: 465mg

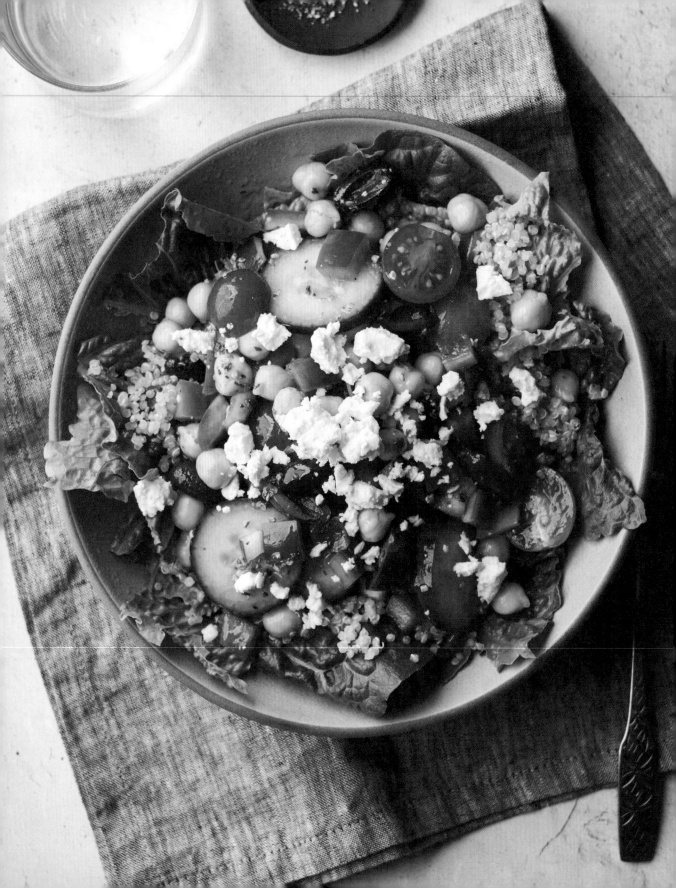

SALADS AND HEALTHY BOWLS

CAPRESE SALAD WITH BALSAMIC GLAZE

Serves 4 to 6 · Prep time: 10 minutes / Cook time: 15 minutes
GLUTEN-FREE, 30 MINUTES OR LESS, VEGETARIAN

Herbs are a great way to add a punch of flavor to meals without adding any empty calories. Both fresh and dried versions are easy to incorporate into many meals like pasta sauces, pizzas, soups, and salads. This salad uses one of my favorite herbs, basil.

2 cups halved grape tomatoes

8 ounces fresh mozzarella cheese, cut into ½-inch cubes

¼ cup chopped fresh basil

2 tablespoons olive oil

1 garlic clove, minced

¼ teaspoon hemp hearts

¼ teaspoon sea salt

⅛ teaspoon freshly ground black pepper

½ cup balsamic vinegar

1. In a large bowl, mix the tomatoes, mozzarella cheese, and basil. Add the olive oil, garlic, hemp hearts, salt, and pepper and stir to combine. Let marinate for 15 minutes.

2. In a saucepan, heat the balsamic vinegar over low heat. Bring it to a simmer and cook until slightly thickened, 7 to 10 minutes.

3. Drizzle the mixture over the salad and serve.

> **SUBSTITUTION TIP:** If you don't have fresh basil on hand, you can use 1 teaspoon of dried basil. Taste and add more if desired.

PER SERVING: Calories: 311; Fat: 20g; Total Carbohydrates: 21g; Net Carbs: 20g; Fiber: 1g; Protein: 13g; Sodium: 481mg

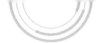

GOAT CHEESE AND SALMON SALAD

Serves 4 · Prep time: 10 minutes / Cook time: 15 minutes
GLUTEN-FREE, 30 MINUTES OR LESS

Say cheese! Yes, you can eat cheese and still achieve your fitness goals. This meal is loaded with protein, but if you require more, increase the portion of salmon, not the cheese. The salmon will increase the amount of healthy fats in this meal.

1 (12-ounce) salmon fillet

½ tablespoon olive oil

½ teaspoon sea salt

¼ teaspoon freshly
   ground black pepper

12 cups fresh
   baby spinach

2 cups sliced strawberries

1 cup diced cucumbers

¼ small red onion,
   thinly sliced

1 medium avocado, pitted,
   peeled, and sliced

½ cup chopped pecans

½ cup crumbled
   goat cheese

3 tablespoons balsamic
   vinegar, plus more
   if desired

1. Preheat the oven to 450° F. Line a baking sheet with aluminum foil.

2. Put the salmon on the prepared baking sheet, brush it with the olive oil, and season with the salt and pepper. Bake for 10 to 12 minutes, or until the salmon is cooked through.

3. While the salmon is baking, combine the spinach, strawberries, cucumbers, red onion, avocado, pecans, and goat cheese in a large bowl. Drizzle with the balsamic vinegar and toss gently until evenly coated.

4. Divide the salad equally between 4 bowls. Cut the salmon into 4 equal pieces and place 1 on each salad. Drizzle with additional balsamic vinegar, if desired, and serve immediately.

> **SUBSTITUTION TIP:** If you don't like pecans, you can replace them with almonds.

PER SERVING: Calories: 422; Fat: 28g; Total Carbohydrates: 21g; Net Carbs: 11g; Fiber: 10g; Protein: 26g; Sodium: 412mg

BLACK BEAN AND CORN
CHICKEN SALAD

Serves 2 · Prep time: 10 minutes / Cook time: 15 minutes
GLUTEN-FREE, NUT-FREE, 30 MINUTES OR LESS

Don't be fooled by the easy preparation time for this meal. It is loaded with fat, protein, and fiber. The main sources of each macronutrient are easy to identify, making it simple to track. If you're looking to increase protein, adjust the chicken breast or black beans, or adjust the olive oil for healthy fats.

2 teaspoons lime juice

2½ teaspoons olive
 oil, divided

½ teaspoon garlic powder

10 ounces boneless, skinless chicken breasts, cut
 into bite-size pieces

Sea salt

Freshly ground
 black pepper

½ cup frozen corn kernels

⅔ cup canned black
 beans, drained
 and rinsed

4 cups mixed greens

½ cup baby tomatoes, halved

2 scallions, green parts
 only, thinly sliced

⅔ cup fat-free sour cream

1. In a small bowl, mix the lime juice, ½ teaspoon of olive oil, and garlic powder. Set aside.

2. In a large nonstick skillet, heat the remaining 2 teaspoons of olive oil over medium-high heat. Add the chicken and cook, stirring occasionally, until golden brown and cooked through, 8 to 11 minutes. Season with salt and pepper to taste. Set aside.

3. While the chicken is cooking, in a small saucepan, cook the frozen corn according to the package instructions. Drain the corn.

4. In a medium bowl, mix the corn, black beans, greens, tomatoes, and scallions. Drizzle with the lime juice dressing and mix again. Divide the mixture equally between 2 bowls and top with the chicken and dollops of sour cream. Season with salt and pepper to taste, and serve immediately.

> **LEFTOVER TIP:** Refrigerate any extra salad in an airtight container and store the sour cream separately. Add sour cream just before serving.

PER SERVING: Calories: 424; Fat: 10g; Total Carbohydrates: 41g; Net Carbs: 32g; Fiber: 9g; Protein: 43g; Sodium: 228mg

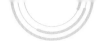

BLACK BEAN BURRITO BOWL

Serves 4 · Prep time: 10 minutes / Cook time: 50 minutes
DAIRY-FREE, GLUTEN-FREE, VEGAN

4 medium sweet potatoes, peeled and cut into 1-inch slices

2 tablespoons olive oil, divided

1 teaspoon chili powder, divided

½ teaspoon sea salt, divided, plus more for seasoning

1 (15-ounce) can black beans

1 teaspoon ground cumin

¼ teaspoon garlic powder

1½ cups quinoa

2 small avocados, sliced

8 tablespoons pepitas

¼ teaspoon freshly ground black pepper

1. Preheat the oven to 425°F. Line a baking sheet with parchment paper.

2. In a large bowl, mix the sweet potatoes, 1 tablespoon of olive oil, ½ teaspoon of chili powder, and ¼ teaspoon of salt until the potatoes are evenly coated. Arrange the sweet potatoes on a baking sheet, making sure not to overcrowd them. Bake for 15 minutes, flip the potatoes, and continue to bake for another 20 to 25 minutes, or until the potatoes are tender.

3. While the potatoes are baking, in a small saucepan, heat the black beans and their liquid over medium-low heat. Add the cumin, garlic powder, and the remaining ¼ teaspoon of salt and simmer until heated through, about 5 minutes. Drain and set aside.

4. Cook the quinoa according to the package instructions. Set aside.

5. To assemble the bowls: Divide the quinoa between 4 bowls. Top each bowl with ¼ of the sweet potatoes, ¼ of the bean mixture, and ¼ of the avocado slices. Sprinkle each bowl with 2 tablespoons of pepitas and season with additional salt and pepper, if desired.

> **COOKING TIP:** It's important to cut the sweet potatoes into 1-inch-thick slices so that they bake evenly. Too thick and they won't crisp properly; too thin, they will burn.

PER SERVING: Calories: 762; Fat: 34g; Total Carbohydrates: 97g; Net Carbs: 73g; Fiber: 24g; Protein: 25g; Sodium: 369mg

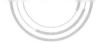

GREEK CHICKPEA POWER BOWL

Serves 4 · Prep time: 10 minutes / Cook time: 30 minutes
GLUTEN-FREE, VEGETARIAN

One of the great things about a basic Greek salad is that you can easily adjust the amounts of protein and even change the type of protein you use. For example, use a cooked chicken breast instead of chickpeas. Need more protein? Double it. Want a less hearty salad? Leave out the chickpeas.

1½ cups quinoa

2 tablespoons red
wine vinegar

2 tablespoons olive oil

1 teaspoon hemp hearts

1 teaspoon dried oregano

1 (15-ounce) can chick-
peas, drained and rinsed

1 cup halved cherry
tomatoes

1 large cucumber, cut into
¼-inch slices

1 large green bell pepper,
seeded and diced

½ medium red
onion, diced

⅓ cup pitted and halved
kalamata olives

4 cups torn
romaine lettuce

½ cup crumbled low-fat
feta cheese

1. Cook the quinoa according to the package instructions.

2. While the quinoa is cooking, in a small bowl, whisk together the red wine vinegar, olive oil, hemp hearts, and oregano. Set aside.

3. In a large bowl, toss together the chickpeas, tomatoes, cucumber, bell pepper, red onion, and kalamata olives. Pour the dressing over the salad and toss until evenly coated.

4. To assemble the bowl, divide the lettuce between 4 bowls. Top with the quinoa and the chickpea mixture. Sprinkle with the feta and serve.

> **SUBSTITUTION TIP:** If you don't have red wine vinegar on hand, you can replace it with lemon juice. And feel free to add sea salt, if desired, though I find that between the feta and olives, not much salt is needed.

PER SERVING: Calories: 477; Fat: 18g; Total Carbohydrates: 65g; Net Carbs: 54g; Fiber: 11g; Protein: 18g; Sodium: 387mg

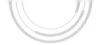

TURMERIC VEGGIE POWER BOWL

Serves 4 · Prep time: 10 minutes / Cook time: 50 minutes
DAIRY-FREE, GLUTEN-FREE, NUT-FREE, VEGAN

This flavorful veggie-loaded bowl can easily be modified to meet your macros.

2 large zucchini, sliced

2 cups halved baby tomatoes

2 tablespoons olive oil, divided

½ teaspoon sea salt

½ teaspoon freshly ground black pepper

3 cups cauliflower florets

½ teaspoon ground cumin

1 teaspoon ground turmeric

1½ cups quinoa

1 cup frozen edamame

1. Preheat the oven to 375°F. Line 2 baking sheets with parchment paper.

2. In a large bowl, mix the zucchini, tomatoes, 1 tablespoon of olive oil, salt, and pepper. In another large bowl, mix the cauliflower, cumin, and turmeric.

3. Spread out the zucchini mixture onto one of the baking sheets. Toss together the cauliflower and remaining 1 tablespoon of olive oil. Spread out the mixture onto the other baking sheet. Avoid overcrowding.

4. Bake the cauliflower for 25 to 30 minutes, or until golden and slightly crisp. Bake the zucchini mixture for 30 to 35 minutes, or until golden and slightly crisp.

5. While the vegetables are baking, cook the quinoa according to package instructions.

6. In a medium pot, combine the edamame and enough water to cover and bring it to a boil over medium-high heat. Cook until tender, 3 to 5 minutes.

7. To assemble the bowls, divide the quinoa equally between 4 bowls. Top with equal amounts of the zucchini mixture, cauliflower, and edamame. Taste and season with additional salt and pepper, if desired.

PER SERVING: Calories: 406; Fat: 14g; Total Carbohydrates: 57g; Net Carbs: 46g; Fiber: 11g; Protein: 17g; Sodium: 280mg

DECONSTRUCTED SUSHI BOWL

Serves 4 · Prep time: 10 minutes / Cook time: 25 minutes
VEGETARIAN

This is one of my favorite bowls to prepare because most of these foods are found in the pantry, refrigerator, or freezer. It's an easy lunch to prep for the week. To maximize flavor without compromising the macronutrient ratio, increase the sriracha or pickled ginger.

2 cups quick brown rice

2 cups shelled edamame

⅛ teaspoon sea salt

1 large cucumber, diced

2 cups fresh or frozen mango pieces

4 tablespoons pickled ginger

2 teaspoons black sesame seeds

4 nori (seaweed) sheets, cut into small pieces

4 tablespoons low-fat mayonnaise

1 teaspoon sriracha

2 tablespoons low-sodium soy sauce

1. Cook the rice according to the package instructions. Set aside.

2. In a medium pot, combine the edamame and enough water to cover and bring it to a boil over medium-high heat. Cook until tender, 3 to 5 minutes. Drain, add the sea salt, and toss until combined.

3. Divide the rice equally between 4 bowls. Top with equal amounts of edamame, cucumber, mango, and pickled ginger. Top with a sprinkle of sesame seeds and the nori pieces.

4. In a small bowl, mix the mayonnaise and sriracha and divide the mixture equally over the 4 bowls. Drizzle the soy sauce over the top and serve.

> **INGREDIENT TIP:** Pickled ginger (sometimes called sushi ginger) can be found in the international aisle of most grocery stores. It can also be purchased online from Save-On-Foods, Walmart, Amazon, and Target.

PER SERVING: Calories: 550; Fat: 11g; Total Carbohydrates: 99g; Net Carbs: 90g; Fiber: 9g; Protein: 18g; Sodium: 294mg

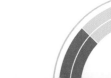

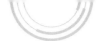

CASHEW CHICKEN BOWL

Serves 4 · Prep time: 10 minutes / Cook time: 30 minutes
DAIRY-FREE

Like many nuts, cashews are calorically dense, so it's important to watch your portion size. If you're looking to reduce or increase the fat content of this meal, adjust or omit the cashews.

1 cup quick brown rice

2 tablespoons
   unsalted cashews

2 tablespoons low-sodium
   soy sauce

2 tablespoons creamy
   100% all-natural
   peanut butter

1 tablespoon maple syrup

½ tablespoon olive oil

3 garlic cloves, minced

1 pound boneless, skin-
   less chicken breast, cut
   into bite-size pieces

Sea salt

Freshly ground
   black pepper

3 scallions, both green
   and white parts, cut into
   diagonal slices

2 cups fresh baby spinach

1. Cook the rice according to the package instructions. Set aside.

2. Put the cashews in a small zip-top plastic bag, seal, and crush them using a rolling pin. Set aside.

3. In a small bowl, mix the soy sauce, peanut butter, and maple syrup. Set aside.

4. In a large nonstick skillet, heat the olive oil over medium-high heat. Add the garlic and sauté for 1 minute. Add the chicken and cook, stirring occasionally, until golden brown and cooked through, 7 to 10 minutes. Season with salt and pepper to taste.

5. Add the cashews and cook for 1 minute. Add the peanut butter mixture and mix well.

6. Reduce the heat to medium-low, add the scallions, and cook, stirring, for another 1 to 2 minutes. Turn off the heat, add the spinach, cover, and let it sit for 2 minutes.

7. Divide the rice equally between 4 bowls, top with the chicken and spinach mixture, and serve immediately.

> **LEFTOVER TIP:** Reheat leftovers in a microwave oven or in a saucepan until heated through and the chicken reaches an internal temperature of 165° F.

PER SERVING: Calories: 424; Fat: 13g; Total Carbohydrates: 45g; Net Carbs: 42g; Fiber: 3g; Protein: 33g; Sodium: 352mg

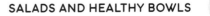

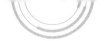

SESAME CHICKEN RICE BOWL

Serves 4 · Prep time: 10 minutes / Cook time: 35 minutes
DAIRY-FREE

These three foods with the rice can be scaled up or down to meet your macro targets: brown rice (complex carbs), chicken (protein), sesame seeds or olive oil (healthy fat).

1½ cups quick brown rice

12 ounces boneless, skinless chicken breast, cut into slices

¼ teaspoon sea salt

⅛ teaspoon freshly ground black pepper

2 tablespoons olive oil, divided

2 red bell peppers, seeded and cut into slices

½ cup rice vinegar

3 scallions, green parts only, thinly sliced

1 tablespoon honey

1 tablespoon low-sodium soy sauce

1 garlic clove, minced

1 tablespoon white sesame seeds

1. Cook the rice according to the package instructions.

2. Season the chicken with the salt and pepper and set aside on a plate.

3. In a large nonstick skillet, heat 1 tablespoon of olive oil over medium heat. Add the peppers and cook, stirring occasionally, until tender, about 10 minutes. Transfer to a bowl and set aside.

4. In the same skillet, heat the remaining 1 tablespoon of olive oil over medium-high heat. Add the chicken and cook, stirring occasionally, until golden brown and cooked through, 7 to 10 minutes. Transfer the chicken to the bowl with the peppers and set aside.

5. To make the sauce, in a small bowl, mix the rice vinegar, scallions, honey, soy sauce, garlic, and sesame seeds. Pour the sauce over the chicken and peppers and mix well until evenly coated.

6. Divide the rice equally between 4 bowls and top with the chicken and bell pepper mixture. Serve immediately.

> **SUBSTITUTION TIP:** You can use quinoa instead of brown rice if you're looking to increase the fiber and protein, both of which can help you feel fuller.

PER SERVING: Calories: 480; Fat: 12g; Total Carbohydrates: 64g; Net Carbs: 60g; Fiber: 4g; Protein: 26g; Sodium: 292mg

SPICY CHICKEN AND RICE BOWL

Serves 4 · Prep time: 10 minutes / Cook time: 40 minutes

DAIRY-FREE

Given that chicken is the main protein macronutrient in this meal, you can adjust the amount to suit your needs. Alternatively, you could adjust the edamame, though this will also impact the carbohydrate content.

1½ cups quick brown rice

1 cup shelled frozen edamame

2 tablespoons creamy 100% all-natural peanut butter

3 tablespoons low-sodium soy sauce

2 teaspoons sriracha

¾ tablespoon plus ½ tablespoon olive oil, divided

3 garlic cloves, minced

18 ounces boneless, skinless chicken breast, cut into bite-size pieces

2 large red bell peppers, seeded and thinly sliced

2 medium carrots, peeled and thinly sliced

4 scallions, thinly sliced, white and green parts separated

1. Cook the brown rice according to the package instructions. In a medium saucepan, combine the edamame and enough water to cover and bring to a boil over medium-high heat. Reduce the heat to medium-low and simmer until tender, 3 to 5 minutes. Drain and set aside.

2. In a small bowl, mix the peanut butter, soy sauce, and sriracha. Set aside.

3. In a large nonstick skillet, heat ¾ tablespoon of olive oil over medium-high heat. Add the garlic and sauté for 1 minute. Add the chicken and cook, stirring often, until golden brown and cooked through, 8 to 12 minutes. Pour the peanut butter sauce over the chicken and mix well. Cover and set aside to keep warm.

4. Warm the remaining ½ tablespoon of olive oil over medium-high heat. Add the bell peppers, carrots, and the white parts of the scallions and cook, stirring occasionally, until tender, 5 to 8 minutes. Add the edamame and sauté for 1 minute. Add the green parts of the scallions and sauté for 1 more minute. Remove from the heat.

5. To assemble the bowls: Divide the rice equally between 4 bowls. Top with the chicken and vegetable mixture and serve immediately.

PER SERVING: Calories: 596; Fat: 16g; Total Carbohydrates: 70g; Net Carbs: 62g; Fiber: 8g; Protein: 43g; Sodium: 501mg

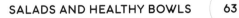

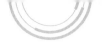

TERIYAKI BEEF AND BROCCOLI BOWL

Serves 4 · Prep time: 10 minutes / Cook time: 35 minutes

DAIRY-FREE, NUT-FREE

2 tablespoons cornstarch

2 cups water, divided

½ cup low-sodium
soy sauce

¼ cup honey

2 teaspoons minced
garlic, divided

2 tablespoons olive
oil, divided

1 pound extra-lean beef,
cut into slices

2 cups broccoli florets

2 scallions, thinly sliced,
white and green parts
separated

Sea salt

1. In a small bowl, mix the cornstarch and ¼ cup of water. Set aside.

2. In a small saucepan, combine the soy sauce, honey, 1 teaspoon of garlic, and 1¾ cups water, and bring it to a boil over medium-high heat. Reduce the heat to low, add the cornstarch and water mixture, and cook, stirring occasionally, until the sauce thickens, 8 to 10 minutes. Set aside.

3. While the sauce is thickening, heat 1 tablespoon of oil in a large nonstick skillet over medium-high heat. Add the beef and cook, stirring occasionally, until browned and cooked through, 8 to 10 minutes. Drain any excess liquid in the pan, transfer the beef to a plate, and set aside.

4. In the same pan, heat the remaining 1 tablespoon of oil over medium-high heat. Add the remaining 1 teaspoon of garlic and sauté for 30 seconds. Add the broccoli and continue to sauté for 3 to 4 minutes. Add the white parts of the scallions and stir to combine. Season with the salt to taste and mix well.

5. Add the beef and thickened sauce to the skillet and stir well.

6. To assemble the bowls, divide the rice equally between 4 bowls. Top with the beef and broccoli mixture and garnish with remaining green parts of the scallions. Serve immediately.

PER SERVING: Calories: 328; Fat: 14g; Total Carbohydrates: 27g; Net Carbs: 25g; Fiber: 2g; Protein: 28g; Sodium: 1262mg

AVOCADO-SALMON POWER BOWL

Serves 4 · Prep time: 10 minutes / Cook time: 55 minutes

DAIRY-FREE, GLUTEN-FREE, NUT-FREE

1½ cups quick brown rice

4 medium sweet potatoes, peeled and cut into 1-inch slices

2½ tablespoons olive oil, divided

½ teaspoon smoked paprika

½ teaspoon sea salt, divided

1 (12-ounce) salmon fillet

½ teaspoon freshly ground black pepper, divided

8 cups spring mix greens

2 small avocados, pitted, peeled, and cut into slices

½ tablespoon freshly squeezed lemon juice

1. Preheat the oven to 425° F. Line 2 baking sheets with parchment paper.

2. Cook the brown rice according to the package instructions and set aside.

3. While the rice is cooking, in a large bowl, mix the sweet potatoes, 2 tablespoons of olive oil, paprika, and ¼ teaspoon of sea salt until evenly coated.

4. Arrange the potato mixture on one of the baking sheets, making sure not to overcrowd. Bake for 20 minutes, flip the potatoes over, and continue to bake for 15 to 20 more minutes, or until the potatoes are tender.

5. While the potatoes are baking, put the salmon on the other baking sheet. Using a basting brush, evenly coat the salmon with the remaining ½ tablespoon of olive oil. Season with the remaining ¼ teaspoon of salt and ¼ teaspoon of pepper. Add the salmon to the oven when the potatoes have 15 minutes left to cook. Check the salmon for doneness after 12 minutes.

6. To assemble the bowls, divide the rice equally between 4 bowls. Top each bowl with the 2 cups of spring mix, ¼ of the avocado slices, 3 ounces of salmon, ¼ of the sweet potatoes, and the lemon juice. Taste and season with the remaining ¼ teaspoon of pepper, as desired.

PER SERVING: Calories: 763; Fat: 31g; Total Carbohydrates: 95g; Net Carbs: 79g; Fiber: 16g; Protein: 29g; Sodium: 353mg

SPICY TUNA POKE BOWL

Serves 4 · Prep time: 10 minutes / Cook time: 30 minutes
DAIRY-FREE

I don't know about you, but I *love* spicy mayo. It adds an extra oomph to meals. The great thing is when you are tracking macros, all the foods fit. To modify the macronutrients, adjust the carbs (the rice), protein (the tuna), and the healthy fat (the avocado).

1½ cups quick brown rice

3 tablespoons low-fat mayonnaise

2 teaspoons sriracha, divided

1 (16-ounce) sashimi-grade tuna fillet, cut into ¾-inch chunks

⅓ cup thinly sliced scallions

3 tablespoons low-sodium soy sauce

2 teaspoons sesame oil

1 tablespoon black sesame seeds, plus more for garnish

2 avocados, pitted, peeled, and sliced

2 red bell peppers, seeded and thinly sliced

1 medium cucumber, cut into ¼-inch slices

1. Cook the rice according to the package instructions. Set aside.

2. In a small bowl, mix the mayonnaise and 1 teaspoon sriracha and set aside.

3. In a medium bowl, gently mix the tuna, scallions, soy sauce, sesame oil, remaining 1 teaspoon of sriracha, and sesame seeds. Set aside for 5 minutes.

4. To assemble the bowls, divide the rice equally between 4 bowls. Top with equal amounts of avocado, bell pepper, and cucumber. Add ¼ of the spicy tuna to each bowl and drizzle with the spicy mayo.

SUBSTITUTION TIP: The add-ins to the bowl can be changed to your liking. For example, to add more vegetables, consider carrots, shredded red cabbage, and radish slices. For extra protein, consider adding edamame.

PER SERVING: Calories: 659; Fat: 24g; Total Carbohydrates: 76g; Net Carbs: 63g; Fiber: 13g; Protein: 39g; Sodium: 459mg

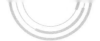

SHRIMP, PEANUT, AND RICE BOWL

Serves 4 · Prep time: 10 minutes / Cook time: 30 minutes

DAIRY-FREE

Peanut butter is a great way to boost the nutritional content of meals, especially the protein and healthy fats. It can easily be incorporated into meals, snacks, and sauces, as in this recipe. It is calorically dense, though, so be careful about portion size.

1½ cups quick brown rice

3 tablespoons low-sodium soy sauce

2 tablespoons creamy 100% all-natural peanut butter

2 teaspoons sriracha

1 tablespoon olive oil

1 cup diced carrots

1 yellow bell pepper, seeded and diced

1 cup thinly sliced mushrooms

4 cups medium shrimp

5 scallions, green parts only, thinly sliced

Sea salt

Freshly ground black pepper

1. Cook the brown rice according to the package instructions. Set aside.

2. In a small bowl, mix the soy sauce, peanut butter, and sriracha. Set aside.

3. Heat the olive oil in a large skillet over medium-high heat. Add the carrots, bell pepper, and mushrooms and cook, stirring occasionally, until tender, for 5 to 7 minutes.

4. Add the shrimp and cook, stirring occasionally, until opaque, 4 to 5 minutes. Remove from the heat, add the sauce, and mix well.

5. To assemble the bowls, divide the rice equally between 4 bowls. Top with the shrimp mixture and garnish with the scallions. Taste and season with the salt and pepper, if desired.

SUBSTITUTION TIP: If you want to make this a gluten-free meal, substitute gluten-free soy sauce.

PER SERVING: Calories: 506; Fat: 12g; Total Carbohydrates: 64g; Net Carbs: 59g; Fiber: 5g; Protein: 36g; Sodium: 1,555mg

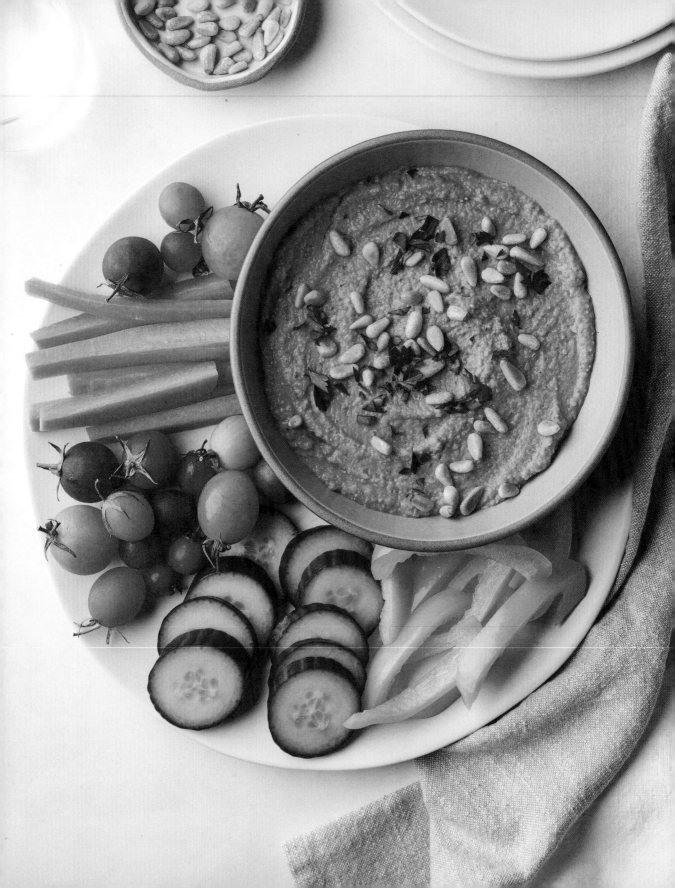

SNACKS, SIDES, DIPS, AND SAUCES

CHILI-CHIVE POPCORN

Serves 4 · Prep time: 5 minutes / Cook time: 10 minutes
DAIRY-FREE, GLUTEN-FREE, NUT-FREE, 30 MINUTES OR LESS, VEGAN

Popcorn has to be one of my most recommended snacks because it's loaded with fiber. In fact, 2 cups of air-popped popcorn provide about 2 grams of fiber and only 60 calories. It also can be paired with a variety of nuts to help increase the healthy fat content.

2½ tablespoons olive oil, divided

½ cup popcorn kernels

½ teaspoon garlic powder

½ teaspoon onion powder

3 tablespoons minced fresh chives

2 tablespoons nutritional yeast

¼ teaspoon sea salt

¼ teaspoon chili flakes (optional)

1. Heat 2 tablespoons of olive oil in a large pot over medium heat. Add the popcorn kernels, cover, and cook, shaking the pot often, until there are 3 seconds between pops and most of the kernels have popped. Transfer the popcorn to a large bowl.

2. Heat the remaining ½ tablespoon of olive oil in a very small saucepan over medium heat. Add the garlic powder and onion powder and cook, stirring constantly, for about 1 minute.

3. Pour the seasoned oil over the popcorn and mix well. Add the chives, nutritional yeast, salt, and chili flakes, if using, and toss until evenly coated.

4. Divide the popcorn equally into 4 bowls.

> **COOKING TIP:** To extract more of the garlic flavor from the powder, mix the garlic powder with ½ teaspoon of water before adding it to the heated oil.

PER SERVING: Calories: 203; Fat: 10g; Total Carbohydrates: 24g; Net Carbs: 19g; Fiber: 5g; Protein: 6g; Sodium: 386mg

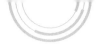

CHEESY PEPPERED KALE CHIPS

Serves 4 · Prep time: 5 minutes / Cook time: 20 minutes
DAIRY-FREE, GLUTEN-FREE, NUT-FREE, 30 MINUTES OR LESS, VEGAN

Even if you're not a huge fan of kale in a salad, I think you'll enjoy these crispy kale chips. There is a reason kale is so popular. It packs in vitamins A, C, and K and calcium while keeping the calories low. Still not convinced? The nutritional yeast in this recipe lends a cheesy flavor, minus the saturated fat. Try it!

6 ounces kale, stemmed, washed, and dried
2 teaspoons olive oil
1½ tablespoons nutritional yeast
¼ teaspoon sea salt
½ teaspoon freshly ground black pepper

1. Preheat the oven to 225° F. Line a baking sheet with parchment paper.

2. In a large bowl, mix the kale and olive oil until evenly coated. Put the kale onto the prepared baking sheet.

3. Sprinkle the nutritional yeast, salt, and pepper over the kale.

4. Bake for 15 minutes, or until the edges of the kale are slightly brown. To increase the crispiness, rotate the pan and continue to bake for another 3 to 5 minutes. Watch closely to avoid burning.

5. Let the kale chips cool on the pan for 2 minutes to increase the crispiness. Transfer to a large bowl and let cool completely before serving.

> **INGREDIENT TIP:** Nutritional yeast adds a savory, Parmesan-like flavor to the popcorn. This power food provides protein, fiber, potassium, and vitamin B_{12}, making it a great addition for those following a vegan or vegetarian diet.

PER SERVING: Calories: 53; Fat: 3g; Total Carbohydrates: 5g; Net Carbs: 3g; Fiber: 2g; Protein: 3g; Sodium: 332mg

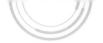

ROASTED EDAMAME WITH EVERYTHING BAGEL SEASONING

Serves 4 · Prep time: 5 minutes, plus 20 minutes drying time /
Cook time: 35 minutes

DAIRY-FREE, GLUTEN-FREE, VEGAN

The combination of ingredients in everything bagel seasoning can pair with many foods besides the beloved breakfast item, including edamame. This recipe can make for an easy on-the-go snack and is loaded with protein.

15 ounces frozen shelled
   edamame, rinsed
   and dried
1 teaspoon white
   sesame seeds
½ teaspoon black
   sesame seeds
½ teaspoon dried garlic
½ teaspoon dried onion
½ teaspoon sea salt
¼ teaspoon poppy seeds
2 teaspoons olive oil

1. Preheat the oven to 375° F. Line a baking sheet with parchment paper.

2. Put the frozen edamame in a colander and quickly run them under warm water to remove any ice. Pat the edamame dry using a clean dish towel and set aside for 20 minutes to dry completely.

3. While the edamame is drying, in a small bowl, mix the white and black sesame seeds, garlic, onion, salt, and poppy seeds.

4. In a large mixing bowl, toss together the dried edamame and olive oil until evenly coated. Add the seasoning mixture and mix well. Spread out the seasoned edamame on the prepared baking sheet. Avoid overcrowding.

5. Roast for 35 to 40 minutes, stirring every 10 minutes, or until crispy. Transfer the edamame to a bowl and serve. Refrigerate any leftovers in an airtight container for up to 3 days.

> **PREP TIP:** The drier the edamame, the crispier they will be. If you have more time to spare, allow the edamame to dry for 30 minutes.

PER SERVING: Calories: 158; Fat: 8g; Total Carbohydrates: 11g; Net Carbs: 5g; Fiber: 6g; Protein: 12g; Sodium: 240mg

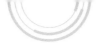

TURMERIC ROASTED CHICKPEAS

Serves 4 · Prep time: 5 minutes, plus 15 minutes drying time /
Cook time: 35 minutes

DAIRY-FREE, GLUTEN-FREE, NUT-FREE, VEGAN

There has been a lot of talk about turmeric lately, and for good reason. Its potential role in the anti-inflammatory process has made it very desirable. Plus, it adds color and an earthy flavor to foods. My advice? Be careful how much turmeric you add and avoid spillage. The powdered variety tends to leave its brilliant-yellow mark behind.

1 (15-ounce) can chick-
   peas, drained and rinsed
½ teaspoon ground
   turmeric
½ teaspoon garlic powder
½ teaspoon sea salt
¼ teaspoon freshly
   ground black pepper
2 teaspoons olive oil

1. Preheat the oven to 375° F. Line a baking sheet with parchment paper.

2. Pat the chickpeas dry with a clean kitchen towel. Spread out the dried chickpeas on the prepared baking sheet. Avoid overcrowding. Let the chickpeas dry for at least 15 minutes.

3. Bake for 30 to 35 minutes, shaking the baking sheet every 10 minutes, or until the chickpeas are a light golden brown.

4. While the chickpeas are baking, in a small bowl, mix the turmeric, garlic powder, salt, and pepper.

5. Transfer the roasted chickpeas to a medium bowl. Add the olive oil and toss until evenly coated. Add the seasoning and toss until evenly coated.

6. Store any leftovers in a container for up to 4 days. Cover loosely to maintain crispiness.

> **PREP TIP:** The drier the chickpeas, the crispier they will be. If you have more time to spare, allow them to dry for 30 minutes.

PER SERVING: Calories: 101; Fat: 4g; Total Carbohydrates: 14g; Net Carbs: 10g; Fiber: 4g; Protein: 4g; Sodium: 354mg

SPICY SNACK MIX

Serves 4 · Prep time: 5 minutes / Cook time: 5 minutes
DAIRY-FREE, 30 MINUTES OR LESS, VEGAN

This spicy snack mix adds more nutrition and kick to the classic party mix, and I think you'll love it. It's easy to prepare and is loaded with fiber and healthy fat.

1 tablespoon reduced-sodium soy sauce

1 tablespoon freshly squeezed lemon juice

⅛ teaspoon onion powder

⅛ teaspoon garlic powder

⅛ teaspoon cayenne pepper

¼ cup raw pepitas

⅓ cup whole almonds

⅓ cup unsalted cashews

½ cup unsalted air-popped popcorn

½ cup unsalted mini pretzel sticks

1. In a small bowl, mix the soy sauce, lemon juice, onion powder, garlic powder, and cayenne pepper. Set aside.

2. In a large skillet over medium-low heat, combine the pepitas, almonds, and cashews and cook, stirring frequently, until toasted, 2 to 3 minutes. Immediately drizzle with the soy sauce mixture and remove the pan from the heat. Add the popcorn and pretzels and stir until evenly coated. Transfer the mixture to a large bowl and serve immediately.

3. Store any leftover snack mix in an airtight container for up to 3 days.

COOKING TIP: Be sure to watch the nuts very carefully when toasting them; they burn easily. To increase the oil in the mix, heat ⅛ to ¼ teaspoon olive oil before adding the pepitas and nuts.

PER SERVING: Calories: 233; Fat: 15g; Total Carbohydrates: 19g; Net Carbs: 16g; Fiber: 3g; Protein: 8g; Sodium: 167mg

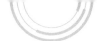

CHEWY BANANA BITES

Makes 12 bites · Prep time: 10 minutes / Cook time: 15 minutes
DAIRY-FREE, 30 MINUTES OR LESS, VEGAN

Ripe bananas are great for baking. They not only add natural sweetness but also help form the base for many baked goods, including these bites. The inclusion of hemp hearts and flaxseed help to increase both the healthy fat and protein content.

¼ cup whole
    unsalted almonds
2 large ripe bananas
1 cup plus 2 tablespoons
    rolled oats
4 teaspoons hemp hearts
2 tablespoons ground
    flaxseed
1 tablespoon
    vanilla extract
2 teaspoons ground
    cinnamon
⅛ teaspoon sea salt
2½ tablespoons 70% dark
    chocolate chips

1. Preheat the oven to 350° F. Line a baking sheet with parchment paper.

2. Put the almonds in a small zip-top plastic bag, seal, and crush them using a rolling pin.

3. In a large bowl, mash the bananas with a fork. Add the oats, hemp hearts, flaxseed, almonds, vanilla, cinnamon, and salt and mix well. Add the chocolate chips and mix until well combined.

4. Using your hands, form the mixture into 12 equal balls and place them on the prepared baking sheet. Using a spoon, gently press down on each ball to flatten the tops.

5. Bake for 15 minutes, or until slightly golden. Let the bites cool on a wire rack for 10 minutes before serving.

6. Store any leftover bites in an airtight container for up to 3 days.

> **SUBSTITUTION TIP:** To make this recipe gluten-free, use gluten-free oats. Be sure to check the package label to ensure oats were processed in a completely gluten-free facility.

PER SERVING (1 BITE): Calories: 95; Fat: 4g; Total Carbohydrates: 13g; Net Carbs: 10g; Fiber: 3g; Protein: 3g; Sodium: 21mg

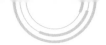

CHOCOLATE–GRAHAM CRACKER CUPS

Makes 6 cups · Prep time: 5 minutes, plus 30 minutes chill time /
Cook time: 10 minutes

NUT-FREE, VEGETARIAN

½ cup pitted dates

1 teaspoon vanilla extract

¼ cup crushed graham
   crackers plus
   1 tablespoon for
   sprinkling

2 tablespoons ground
   flaxseed

1 teaspoon maple syrup

1 cup nonfat plain
   Greek yogurt

1 tablespoon 70% dark
   chocolate chips

1. Line a 6-cup muffin tin with liners. Set aside.

2. In a small bowl, soak the dates in hot water for
    10 minutes. Drain well.

3. In a food processor, combine the soaked dates
    and vanilla and pulse until it forms a jamlike
    consistency. You may need to stop and scrape
    down the sides with a rubber spatula a few times.
    Transfer the mixture to a large bowl.

4. Add ¼ cup of graham crumbles, ground flaxseed,
    and maple syrup and stir until combined. Divide
    the mixture equally among the muffin cups and
    press it down to form a crust. Divide the Greek
    yogurt equally over the crust.

5. In a microwave-safe bowl, microwave the choc-
    olate chips for 25 seconds, stir, and microwave
    again for 25 seconds. Continue to do this until the
    chocolate is melted and smooth.

6. Using a spoon, quickly drizzle the chocolate
    over the muffin cups. Sprinkle the remaining
    1 tablespoon graham crumble over the cups.
    Freeze the pan for at least 30 minutes.

7. When ready to eat, let the graham cracker cups sit
    at room temperature for 5 minutes before serving.

8. Freeze any leftover cups in an airtight container,
    using parchment paper to separate them if
    needed, for up to 2 weeks.

PER SERVING (1 CUP): Calories: 147; Fat: 3g; Total Carbohydrates: 23g;
Net Carbs: 20g; Fiber: 3g; Protein: 8g; Sodium: 49mg

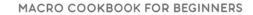

OATMEAL AND RAISIN ENERGY BAR

Makes 6 bars · Prep time: 10 minutes / Cook time: 25 minutes
DAIRY-FREE

The difference between purchasing energy bars and making them yourself is that you know exactly what ingredients are being used, and they taste delicious. As an added bonus, you can modify the ingredients. The combination of oats and almonds provides fiber that helps with fullness.

1 cup rolled oats

½ cup plus 2 tablespoons unsweetened applesauce

2 teaspoons vanilla extract

3 tablespoons whole unsalted almonds

3 tablespoons dark chocolate chips

2 tablespoons pepitas

2 tablespoons raisins

⅛ teaspoon sea salt

1. Preheat the oven to 350° F. Line a small baking pan or a mini loaf pan with parchment paper.

2. In a large bowl, mix the oats, applesauce, and vanilla. Add the almonds, chocolate chips, pepitas, raisins, and salt and mix until combined. Spoon the mixture into the prepared pan and spread it out evenly.

3. Bake for 22 to 25 minutes, or until golden brown around the edges. Let cool completely on a wire rack. Using a knife, loosen the edges and cut into 6 bars. Serve immediately.

> **PREP TIP:** Choose unsalted nuts and seeds. Then you can adjust the salt to your liking.

PER SERVING (1 BAR): Calories: 154; Fat: 7g; Total Carbohydrates: 19g; Net Carbs: 16g; Fiber: 3g; Protein: 5g; Sodium: 54mg

POWER COOKIES

Makes 8 cookies · Prep time: 10 minutes / Cook time: 15 minutes
DAIRY-FREE, 30 MINUTES OR LESS, VEGETARIAN

Confession: I love cookies, and I love baking them even more. And that's because l love the smell of cookies baking in the oven. I've added ingredients like oats to increase the fiber content, which can keep hunger at bay. Maple syrup and dark chocolate can satiate that sweet tooth.

1 cup rolled oats

½ cup oat flour

1 teaspoon ground cinnamon

1 teaspoon baking powder

⅛ teaspoon sea salt

1½ tablespoons melted coconut oil

¼ cup maple syrup

1 large egg, beaten

1 tablespoon vanilla extract

2 tablespoons pepitas

2 tablespoons dark chocolate chips

1. Preheat the oven to 350° F. Line a baking sheet with parchment paper.

2. In a large bowl, mix the oats, oat flour, cinnamon, baking powder, and salt.

3. In a small bowl, mix the coconut oil, maple syrup, egg, and vanilla.

4. Add the wet ingredients to the dry ingredients and mix until combined. Add the pepitas and chocolate chips and mix until combined.

5. Using your hands, form the mixture into 8 balls and place them on the prepared baking sheet. Using a spoon, flatten the tops.

6. Bake for 10 to 12 minutes, or until golden brown. Let the cookies cool on the baking sheet for 3 minutes. Transfer the cookies to a wire rack and let cool completely.

7. Store leftover cookies in an airtight container for up to 3 days.

> **SUBSTITUTION TIP:** Don't have oat flour? That's okay. Use a food processor to grind rolled oats into flour. You can grind more than you need and keep it for future use.

PER SERVING (1 COOKIE): Calories: 158; Fat: 6g; Total Carbohydrates: 21g; Net Carbs: 19g; Fiber: 2g; Protein: 4g; Sodium: 51mg

BAKED PARMESAN CAULIFLOWER

Cauliflower has celebrity status among cruciferous vegetables. Why? Because this versatile vegetable can be turned into "rice" and pizza crust or enjoyed raw. This recipe makes a great side for Pesto Chicken (**page 119**) or Baked Salmon with Green Beans (**page 122**).

4 cups cauliflower florets

1½ tablespoons olive oil

2 teaspoons lemon juice

1½ teaspoons garlic powder

½ teaspoon sea salt

¼ teaspoon freshly ground black pepper

⅓ cup grated reduced-fat Parmesan cheese

1. Preheat the oven to 400° F. Line a baking sheet with parchment paper.

2. In a large bowl, toss the cauliflower with the olive oil and lemon juice. Add the garlic powder, salt, and pepper and mix until combined. Spread the cauliflower on the prepared baking sheet. Pour any remaining seasoning over the cauliflower.

3. Bake for 18 to 20 minutes, or until the cauliflower is golden and crispy. Sprinkle with the Parmesan cheese and continue to bake for 2 to 3 more minutes, or until the cheese has melted. Serve immediately.

> **SUBSTITUTION TIP:** Broccoli makes a good substitute here, and if you want it to be cheesier, increase the Parmesan cheese, but be careful of portion control.

PER SERVING: Calories: 98; Fat: 7g; Total Carbohydrates: 6g; Net Carbs: 4g; Fiber: 2g; Protein: 4g; Sodium: 392mg

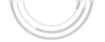

SAUTÉED SPINACH WITH GARLIC AND SESAME

Serves 2 · Prep time: 5 minutes / Cook time: 5 minutes
DAIRY-FREE, GLUTEN-FREE, 30 MINUTES OR LESS, VEGAN

Taking its inspiration from Japanese cooking, this super-simple sautéed spinach with garlic and sesame makes a bold and healthy side dish. It pairs wonderfully with salmon, chicken, and much more.

½ tablespoon white
   sesame seeds
½ tablespoon olive oil
1 garlic clove, minced
8 cups fresh baby spinach
⅛ teaspoon freshly
   squeezed lemon juice

1. Heat a nonstick skillet over medium heat. Add the sesame seeds and cook them until toasted, 3 to 4 minutes. Pay close attention so they don't burn. Once toasted, remove from heat and set aside.

2. Heat the oil in the same skillet over medium heat. Add the garlic and sauté until the color slightly changes, about 1 minute. Turn off the heat, add the spinach, and mix well. Cover with a lid and let sit until the spinach slightly wilts, about 2 minutes.

3. Remove the pan from the heat, add the lemon juice, and stir until combined. Garnish with the toasted sesame seeds and serve.

> **PREP TIP:** Consider using a garlic press to crush the garlic. It's a little faster and delivers the same delicious flavor.

PER SERVING: Calories: 36; Fat: 3g; Total Carbohydrates: 3g; Net Carbs: 1g; Fiber: 2g; Protein: 2g; Sodium: 48mg

CREAMY SPINACH–STUFFED MUSHROOMS

Serves 4 • Prep time: 10 minutes / Cook time: 20 minutes
GLUTEN-FREE, NUT-FREE, 30 MINUTES OR LESS, VEGETARIAN

If you're looking to add some flavor to your vegetables, this recipe is for you. If you don't love vegetables but want to cut back on meat, this recipe accomplishes that. The firm texture of mushrooms mimics meat, making it a delicious substitution or a great side or yummy snack.

Nonstick cooking spray

12 large button
  mushrooms

½ cup low-fat French
  onion dip or sour cream

2 tablespoons low-fat
  cream cheese

1 cup chopped
  fresh spinach

Sea salt

Freshly ground
  black pepper

1. Preheat the oven to 375° F. Lightly spray a 12-cup muffin tin with nonstick cooking spray.

2. Cut the stems off the mushrooms, chop them up, and set them aside.

3. In a bowl, mix the French onion dip and cream cheese. Add the spinach and chopped mushroom stalks and stir to combine. Season with the salt and pepper, if desired.

4. Place 1 mushroom cap, top-down, in each muffin cup. Spoon the mixture equally into each mushroom cap.

5. Bake for 12 minutes. Set the oven to broil and broil for 2 to 3 minutes, until the stuffed mushrooms are browned and heated through. Serve immediately.

> **INGREDIENT TIP:** Choose low-fat options of the French onion dip or sour cream to help reduce saturated fat and calories. To add more flavor, add some onion powder into the spinach mixture.

PER SERVING: Calories: 84; Fat: 5g; Total Carbohydrates: 5g; Net Carbs: 4g; Fiber: 1g; Protein: 5g; Sodium: 95mg

SMASHED POTATOES

Serves 4 · Prep time: 25 minutes / Cook time: 20 minutes
DAIRY-FREE, GLUTEN-FREE, NUT-FREE, VEGAN

Hot potatoes (literally) coming through! Yes, you can eat potatoes and still hit your weight goals. And, no, you don't have to "restrict" other carbs. All foods fit, but it's a matter of finding a portion that works for you. What often lands potatoes in trouble are the toppings like sour cream or gravy.

2 pounds Yukon Gold potatoes, boiled

Nonstick cooking spray

1½ tablespoons olive oil

½ tablespoon chopped fresh parsley

½ tablespoon dried thyme

½ teaspoon garlic powder

¼ teaspoon sea salt

¼ teaspoon freshly ground black pepper

1. Put the potatoes in a large pot and cover them with water. Bring the pot to a boil over high heat and cook until tender, about 15 minutes.

2. Preheat the oven to broil. Lightly spray a baking sheet with nonstick cooking spray.

3. Arrange the potatoes on the prepared baking sheet. Using the bottom of a mason jar or other flat surface, lightly flatten the potatoes—do not mash.

4. Using a small basting brush, brush the olive oil over the potatoes.

5. In a small bowl, mix the parsley, thyme, garlic powder, salt, and pepper. Sprinkle the seasoning evenly over the potatoes. Lightly spray the potatoes with nonstick cooking spray.

6. Broil for 10 to 15 minutes, or until golden and crispy.

> **PREP TIP:** You can boil the potatoes ahead of time and have them ready to broil, which will make this ready much faster. To cook the potatoes, put them in a large pot of salted water and bring to a boil. Cook for 30 to 35 minutes or until fork-tender. Drain.

PER SERVING: Calories: 225; Fat: 5g; Total Carbohydrates: 41g; Net Carbs: 38g; Fiber: 3g; Protein: 5g; Sodium: 157mg

EGGPLANT BITES WITH ZESTY GARLIC MAYO

Serves 4 · Prep time: 20 minutes / Cook time: 25 minutes
GLUTEN-FREE, NUT-FREE, VEGETARIAN

Yes, yes, I know, most people do not like eggplant. I didn't, either, until I figured out a fun way to serve them. When eggplant is baked until it becomes crispy, it turns into a fun dipping vegetable. They're a good source of fiber and potassium and low in calories—a great way to add volume to a meal or snack. Plus, they taste great.

Nonstick cooking spray
1 (15-ounce) eggplant,
  ends trimmed and cut
  into ½-inch slices
½ teaspoon sea salt
1½ tablespoons olive oil
½ teaspoon garlic powder
¼ teaspoon freshly
  ground black pepper
½ cup low-fat mayonnaise
½ cup nonfat plain
  Greek yogurt
2 garlic cloves, crushed
1 tablespoon lemon zest

1. Preheat the oven to 350° F. Lightly spray a baking sheet with nonstick cooking spray.

2. Arrange the eggplant slices on the prepared baking sheet and sprinkle with the salt. Let sit for 15 minutes. Gently pat the eggplant slices dry with paper towels.

3. Using a small basting brush, brush olive oil on each slice. Sprinkle with garlic powder and pepper.

4. Bake for 25 minutes, rotating the baking sheet after 15 minutes, until browned and crispy.

5. While eggplant bites are baking, in a small bowl, mix the mayonnaise, yogurt, garlic, and lemon zest.

6. Serve the eggplant bites hot with the garlic mayonnaise on the side for dipping.

> **PREP TIP:** If you have time, let the eggplant slices sit for 30 minutes so they release more water. This will help increase the final crispiness of the eggplant bites.

PER SERVING: Calories: 166; Fat: 11g; Total Carbohydrates: 14g; Net Carbs: 10g; Fiber: 4g; Protein: 5g; Sodium: 278mg

TURKEY BACON–WRAPPED ASPARAGUS

Serves 4 or 5 · Prep time: 10 minutes / Cook time: 20 minutes
GLUTEN-FREE, NUT-FREE, 30 MINUTES OR LESS

Turkey bacon–wrapped asparagus makes an impressive yet simple side dish or snack, especially if you want a low-carb treat to balance out your macros for the day. Asparagus is a superfood, containing important nutrients like folate and vitamin C.

Nonstick cooking spray

20 asparagus spears, ends trimmed

10 slices reduced-fat turkey bacon, each halved lengthwise

¼ teaspoon sea salt

¼ teaspoon freshly ground black pepper

¼ cup grated reduced-fat Parmesan cheese

1. Preheat the oven to 400° F. Spray a baking sheet with nonstick cooking spray.

2. Take 1 asparagus spear and wrap it with 1 slice of turkey bacon and place it on the prepared baking sheet. Repeat with the remaining asparagus. Sprinkle with the salt and pepper.

3. Bake for 18 to 20 minutes, or until crispy. Sprinkle with the Parmesan cheese and bake for 1 more minute, or until the cheese melts. Serve warm.

> **SUBSTITUTION TIP:** You can omit the cheese or try a different variety, such as smoked Gouda.

PER SERVING: Calories: 107; Fat: 7g; Total Carbohydrates: 4g; Net Carbs: 2g; Fiber: 2g; Protein: 9g; Sodium: 652mg

GOAT CHEESE AND HEMP SPINACH DIP

Serves 4 · Prep time: 15 minutes / Cook time: 30 minutes
GLUTEN-FREE, VEGETARIAN

Spinach dip is typically higher in fat and calories when it has sour cream and mayonnaise. Using nonfat plain Greek yogurt instead not only provides creaminess and reduces the fat but also increases the protein content.

1 teaspoon olive oil

2 garlic cloves, minced

3 scallions, green parts only, thinly sliced

1 tablespoon hemp hearts

¼ teaspoon dried oregano

¼ teaspoon sea salt

2 cups chopped fresh baby spinach

½ cup nonfat plain Greek yogurt

1 tablespoon 1% milk

2 tablespoons crumbled reduced-fat goat cheese

3 ounces shredded reduced-fat mozzarella cheese, divided

1. Preheat the oven to 375° F.

2. Heat the olive oil in a large nonstick skillet over medium heat. Add the garlic and scallions and cook until tender, 1 to 2 minutes. Add the hemp hearts, oregano, and salt and cook until well blended, another 1 to 2 minutes.

3. Stir in the spinach and cook until heated through, about 2 minutes. Remove from the heat, add the Greek yogurt, milk, goat cheese, and 2 ounces of the mozzarella cheese and stir to combine.

4. Transfer the mixture to a baking dish and bake for 15 to 20 minutes, or until the cheese has melted.

5. Top with the remaining 1 ounce of mozzarella cheese and serve immediately.

LEFTOVER TIP: Although this dip tastes best freshly made, leftovers can be refrigerated in an airtight container for up to 2 days. Reheat in the microwave for 1 minute or in a pan over low heat until heated through.

PER SERVING: Calories: 104; Fat: 6g; Total Carbohydrates: 4g; Net Carbs: 3g; Fiber: 1g; Protein: 10g; Sodium: 291mg

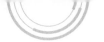

GARLIC–JALAPEÑO GUACAMOLE

Serves 4 · Prep time: 5 minutes / Cook time: 5 minutes

GLUTEN-FREE, NUT-FREE, 30 MINUTES OR LESS, VEGETARIAN

While avocados are technically a fruit, they are loaded with healthy fat. Portion size is important with these because large amounts can greatly impact the macronutrient ratio. Mixing it with nonfat plain Greek yogurt adds creaminess and protein and helps balance the macronutrients.

1 avocado, pitted
  and peeled

¼ cup nonfat plain
  Greek yogurt

¼ medium white
  onion, chopped

1 tablespoon chopped
  fresh cilantro

3 garlic cloves, peeled

1½ tablespoons
  lemon juice

1 teaspoon minced
  jalapeño pepper

¼ teaspoon sea salt

Freshly ground
  black pepper

1. In a food processor, combine the avocado, Greek yogurt, onion, cilantro, garlic, lemon juice, jalapeño, salt, and pepper and puree until smooth.

2. Transfer the mixture to a bowl and serve with baked tortilla chips or vegetables.

> **PREP TIP:** Rinse the avocados thoroughly before cutting into them. Dirt from the skin can transfer to the knife, which can then transfer to the flesh.

PER SERVING: Calories: 108; Fat: 8g; Total Carbohydrates: 8g; Net Carbs: 4g; Fiber: 4g; Protein: 4g; Sodium: 124mg

SPICY RED PEPPER HUMMUS

Serves 6 · Prep time: 10 minutes / Cook time: 20 minutes
DAIRY-FREE, GLUTEN-FREE, VEGAN

Hummus is a wonderfully healthy dip that goes perfectly with raw vegetables. This recipe contains protein, fiber, and healthy fat, and it's loaded with flavor. It's also filling and can be easily adjusted to match your macronutrient ratio.

1 red bell pepper, halved and seeded

2 tablespoons pine nuts

1 (15-ounce) can chickpeas, drained and rinsed

3 garlic cloves, peeled

2 tablespoons olive oil

2 tablespoons lemon juice

1 tablespoon hemp hearts

½ teaspoon chili powder

¼ teaspoon ground cumin

½ teaspoon sea salt

1 tablespoon water

½ tablespoon finely chopped fresh parsley

1. Preheat the broiler. Line a baking sheet with aluminum foil.

2. Place the pepper, cut-side down, on the prepared sheet. Broil for 8 to 10 minutes, or until the skin softens and turns black in spots. Let sit for 5 minutes. When cool enough to handle, peel off the skin and cut the pepper into bite-size pieces.

3. While the pepper is broiling, toast the pine nuts in a nonstick skillet over medium-low heat until golden, 2 to 4 minutes.

4. Puree the red bell pepper, chickpeas, garlic, olive oil, lemon juice, hemp hearts, chili powder, cumin, salt, and 1 tablespoon of water in a food processor until smooth. If needed, add 1 to 2 tablespoons of water to reach the desired consistency.

5. Transfer the mixture to a bowl and garnish with the pine nuts and parsley.

> **LEFTOVER TIP:** Place any remaining hummus in an airtight container and refrigerate for up to 4 days.

PER SERVING: Calories: 103; Fat: 6g; Total Carbohydrates: 11g; Net Carbs: 8g; Fiber: 3g; Protein: 3g; Sodium: 244mg

BLACK BEAN SALSA

Serves 4 · Prep time: 5 minutes / Refrigeration time: 30 minutes
DAIRY-FREE, GLUTEN-FREE, VEGAN

Depending on the ingredients that are added to salsa, it can count toward the total vegetable intake for the day. The addition of black beans increases the protein and fiber content. Add the salsa to nachos or tacos or enjoy it with plain tortilla chips.

1 cup canned black beans, drained and rinsed

1 cup cherry tomatoes, each cut into quarters

⅓ cup diced white onion

½ tablespoon hemp hearts

1 tablespoon olive oil

1 tablespoon freshly squeezed lime juice

¼ teaspoon freshly ground black pepper

⅓ cup chopped fresh cilantro

In a large bowl, mix the black beans, tomatoes, onion, hemp hearts, olive oil, lime juice, pepper, and cilantro. Refrigerate for at least 30 minutes before serving.

> **PREP TIP:** Canned black beans are already cooked, so they are a convenient way to add protein to meals and snacks. Rinse the black beans before using them to reduce the sodium. Refrigerate unused portions in an airtight container for up to 5 days.

PER SERVING: Calories: 100; Fat: 4g; Total Carbohydrates: 13g; Net Carbs: 8g; Fiber: 5g; Protein: 4g; Sodium: 4mg

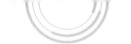

CASHEW PESTO

Serves 6 · Prep time: 5 minutes / Cook time: 10 minutes
GLUTEN-FREE, 30 MINUTES OR LESS

Pesto is well known for its healthy fat content and for adding punches of herby flavor. It can be used in a variety of dishes, including pizza, pasta, salads, and even marinades. Given that it is high in fat, it also is calorically dense, so pay close attention to portion size.

⅓ cup unsalted cashews

1 cup chopped fresh basil

¼ cup olive oil

3 tablespoons grated reduced-fat Parmesan cheese

2 tablespoons lemon juice

1 garlic clove, peeled

½ tablespoon hemp hearts

Sea salt

Freshly ground black pepper

1. Toast the cashews in a nonstick skillet over medium heat for 2 to 3 minutes, or until golden brown.

2. In a food processor, combine the cashews, basil, olive oil, Parmesan cheese, lemon juice, garlic, hemp hearts, salt, and pepper and puree until almost smooth.

3. Store the pesto in an airtight container and refrigerate for up to 1 week.

> **COOKING TIP:** To make the pesto cheesier, increase the cheese by 2 tablespoons. To add spice, replace 1 tablespoon of olive oil with 1 tablespoon of chili oil, ½ teaspoon of chili flakes, or ½ teaspoon of chili powder.

PER SERVING: Calories: 132; Fat: 13g; Total Carbohydrates: 3g; Net Carbs: 3g; Fiber: 0g; Protein: 2g; Sodium: 40mg

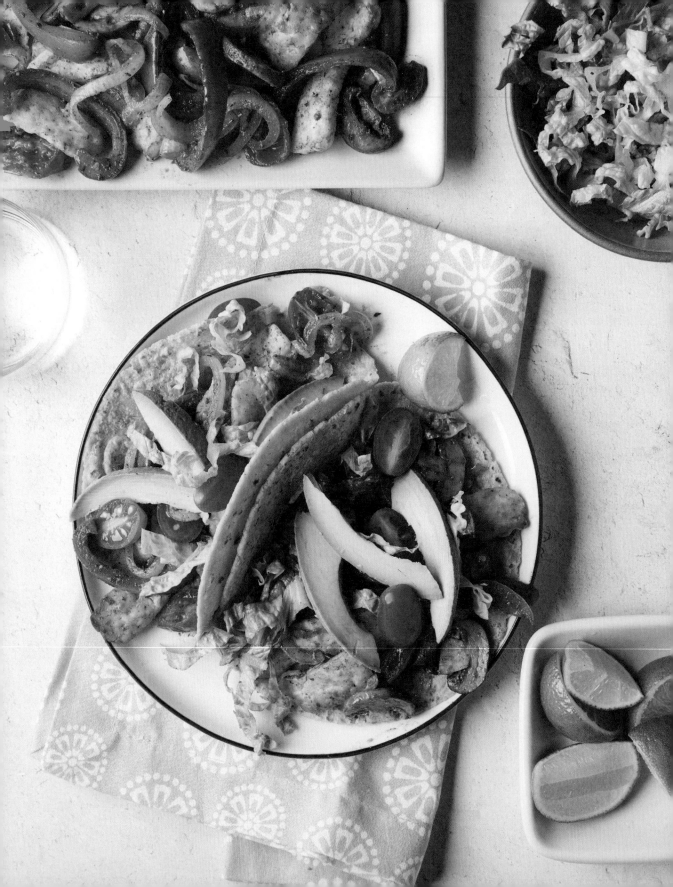

CHAPTER SEVEN

VEGETARIAN MAINS

· · · · · · · · · · · · · · · · · · · ·

WHITE BEAN NACHOS

Serves 4 · Prep time: 10 minutes / Cook time: 10 minutes

NUT–FREE, 30 MINUTES OR LESS, VEGETARIAN

I'm all for eating more plant-based meals, so I thought why not take a classic dish and make it meatless? The easy thing about nachos is that you can pretty much load it up with any vegetable you want. I love adding diced tomatoes or some homemade salsa.

4 ounces unsalted corn tortilla chips

½ tablespoon olive oil

1 green bell pepper, seeded and diced

1 (15-ounce) can low-sodium white beans, drained and rinsed

½ tablespoon taco seasoning

1 teaspoon tomato paste

1 tablespoon water

2 tablespoons all-purpose flour

⅓ cup 1% milk

½ cup shredded low-fat cheddar cheese

2 scallions, green parts only, finely chopped

1. Arrange the tortilla chips on a large plate and set aside.

2. Heat the oil in a large nonstick skillet over medium heat. Add the bell pepper and sauté until tender, 5 to 7 minutes.

3. Add the beans, taco seasoning, tomato paste, and 1 tablespoon of water and cook, stirring occasionally, until heated through. Remove from the heat and set aside.

4. In a small bowl, whisk together the flour and milk.

5. Melt the cheese in a small saucepan over medium-low heat. Add the milk and flour mixture and cook, stirring constantly, until thickened, 1 to 2 minutes. Remove from the heat.

6. Spoon the bean mixture over the tortilla chips, top with the cheese mixture, and sprinkle with the scallions. Serve immediately.

> **SUBSTITUTION TIP:** If you don't like white beans, try black beans or even cooked extra-lean ground chicken.

PER SERVING: Calories: 349; Fat: 12g; Total Carbohydrates: 46g; Net Carbs: 39g; Fiber: 7g; Protein: 15g; Sodium: 378mg

HALLOUMI FAJITAS

Serves 4 · Prep time: 10 minutes / Cook time: 20 minutes
NUT-FREE, 30 MINUTES OR LESS, VEGETARIAN

Fajitas are one of the easiest things to put together—you can cook up everything in one pan or even put it in the oven. To increase the protein content, consider loading up the fajitas with seasoned black beans or chicken. To increase the healthy fat, consider adding slices of avocado or a spoonful of guacamole.

1 green bell pepper, seeded and cut into slices

1 cup sliced grape tomatoes, divided

½ cup sliced mushrooms

⅓ small white onion, thinly sliced

7 ounces Halloumi, cut into strips

½ tablespoon olive oil

1 tablespoon fajita seasoning

8 (6-inch) corn tortillas

2 cups shredded lettuce

1. Preheat the oven to 450° F, line a large baking sheet with parchment paper, and set aside.

2. In a large bowl, add the bell pepper, ½ cup of tomatoes, mushrooms, onion, Halloumi, and olive oil and mix well. Sprinkle with the fajita seasoning, mix again, then arrange on the parchment paper, ensuring it is not overcrowded.

3. Bake in the oven for 12 to 15 minutes, or until golden brown. Remove the cooked Halloumi and continue to cook the vegetables for 5 minutes or until slightly tender.

4. To assemble, evenly divide the filling mixture into the tortillas and top with lettuce and the remaining ½ cup of tomatoes.

> **INGREDIENT TIP:** Halloumi is a salty semihard cheese that has a high melting point, allowing it to retain its shape even after cooking. Oven temperatures can vary, so make sure to check on the Halloumi at 12 minutes. For a crispier texture, allow it to bake for 15 minutes.

PER SERVING: Calories: 346; Fat: 17g; Total Carbohydrates: 32g; Net Carbs: 28g; Fiber: 4g; Protein: 18g; Sodium: 200mg

PARMESAN–CHICKPEA ROTINI

Serves 4 · Prep time: 10 minutes / Cook time: 25 minutes
NUT–FREE, VEGETARIAN

Chickpeas can easily change a classic meal into a meatless one. To make it more complete, pair it with a green salad drizzled with balsamic vinegar.

8 ounces whole-grain rotini

1 (15-ounce) can chickpeas, drained, rinsed, and dried

1½ tablespoons olive oil, divided

3 tablespoons bread crumbs

1½ tablespoons dried oregano, divided

2 teaspoons Italian seasoning, divided

1 large shallot, minced

4 garlic cloves, minced

1 cup canned crushed tomatoes

½ cup 1% milk

2 teaspoons balsamic vinegar

½ cup grated reduced-fat Parmesan cheese

1. Preheat the oven to 375° F. Line a baking sheet with parchment paper.

2. Cook the rotini according to the package instructions. Drain and set aside.

3. In a large bowl, mix the chickpeas, 1 tablespoon of olive oil, the bread crumbs, 1 tablespoon of the oregano, and 1 teaspoon of the Italian seasoning. Spread out the chickpeas on the prepared baking sheet. Avoid overcrowding. Bake for 20 minutes, or until lightly golden. Let cool on the baking sheet on a wire rack.

4. While the chickpeas are in the oven, heat the remaining ½ tablespoon of olive oil in a nonstick skillet over medium heat. Add the shallot and sauté until tender. Add the garlic and sauté until golden, about 1 minute.

5. Add the crushed tomatoes, milk, balsamic vinegar, the remaining ½ tablespoon oregano, and 1 teaspoon Italian seasoning and cook, stirring occasionally, for 1 to 2 minutes. Reduce the heat to low and cook, stirring occasionally, until the sauce slightly thickens, about 4 minutes. Remove from the heat and stir in the chickpeas.

6. Divide the rotini equally between 4 bowls. Top with the chickpea mixture, sprinkle with the Parmesan cheese, and serve immediately.

PER SERVING: Calories: 407; Fat: 11g; Total Carbohydrates: 66g; Net Carbs: 56g; Fiber: 10g; Protein: 17g; Sodium: 438mg

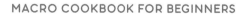

SUN-DRIED TOMATO AND CHICKPEA BOWL

Serves 4 · Prep time: 10 minutes / Cook time: 30 minutes

NUT-FREE, VEGETARIAN

This meal has simple, flavorful, and fiber written all over it. The combination of quinoa and seasoned chickpeas leaves you nothing but full and satisfied. Rinsing chickpeas under cold water may help produce less gas and make them easier to digest. It's also a good way to reduce any added sodium.

1½ cups quinoa

1 (15-ounce) can chickpeas, drained and rinsed

1 teaspoon olive oil

¾ teaspoon garlic powder

¼ teaspoon chili flakes

3 cups fresh baby spinach

4 teaspoons all-purpose flour

1 cup 1% milk

2 tablespoons chopped sun-dried tomatoes

½ cup grated reduced-fat Parmesan cheese

Sea salt to taste

Freshly ground black pepper to taste

1. Cook the quinoa according to the package instructions. Drain and set aside.

2. Put the chickpeas into a large saucepan, add enough water to cover them, and cook over medium heat until heated through, 5 to 10 minutes. Drain the chickpeas and set aside.

3. Heat the olive oil in a large nonstick skillet over medium heat. Add the garlic powder and chili flakes and cook for 30 seconds. Add the spinach and cook, stirring frequently, until it wilts.

4. In a small bowl, whisk together the flour and milk. Reduce the heat to medium-low, add the flour and milk mixture, and cook, stirring, until combined.

5. Add the chickpeas and sun-dried tomatoes and cook, stirring, until thickened, 2 to 4 minutes. Remove from the heat. Add the quinoa and Parmesan and stir until combined. Add the salt and pepper to taste.

6. Divide the mixture equally between 4 bowls and enjoy.

PER SERVING: Calories: 414; Fat: 11g; Total Carbohydrates: 61g; Net Carbs: 52g; Fiber: 9g; Protein: 19g; Sodium: 364mg

HONEY-GARLIC TOFU
AND ASPARAGUS

Serves 4 · **Prep time: 10 minutes / Cook time: 20 minutes**
DAIRY-FREE, NUT-FREE, 30 MINUTES OR LESS

I love making my own sauces so I can control the ingredients. But if you don't have time for that, you can use a store-bought version. Avoid choosing a sauce containing preservatives and high-fructose corn syrup. If you're looking to make this meal gluten-free, be sure to read the label to ensure the soy sauce is processed in a completely gluten-free facility. You'd be surprised how many foods include wheat.

1 (14-ounce) package extra-firm tofu, drained and pressed for 20 minutes

1½ tablespoons olive oil, divided

4 tablespoons cornstarch, divided

12 asparagus spears, trimmed and cut into bite-size pieces

1 cup chopped mushrooms

½ cup low-sodium soy sauce

3 tablespoons honey

1 teaspoon minced fresh ginger

2 teaspoons minced garlic

4 scallions, green parts only, finely chopped

1. Cut the tofu into ½-inch pieces. In a large bowl, toss the tofu with ½ tablespoon of olive oil. Add 2 tablespoons of cornstarch and toss until evenly combined.

2. Heat ½ tablespoon of olive oil in a large nonstick skillet over medium-high heat. Add the tofu and cook, flipping the tofu every 2 to 3 minutes, until slightly browned, 8 to 10 minutes total. Transfer to a bowl and set aside.

3. In the same skillet, heat the remaining ½ tablespoon of oil over medium heat. Add the asparagus and cook for 5 to 6 minutes. Add the mushrooms and cook for 1 minute. Remove the pan from the heat.

4. While the asparagus is cooking, in a small saucepan, combine the soy sauce, honey, ginger, garlic, and ¾ cup water and bring to a boil over medium-high heat.

5. In a small bowl, mix the remaining 2 tablespoons of cornstarch and 1¼ cups of water. Add it to the sauce and mix well. Reduce the heat to low and cook until it reaches the desired thickness, 8 to 10 minutes. Remove from the heat.

6. Add the tofu to the asparagus, pour in the sauce, and stir well.

7. Divide the mixture equally between 4 bowls and garnish with the scallions. Serve immediately.

PREP TIP: To press tofu, wrap it in several layers of paper towel and place it between 2 plates. Place a weight on top and let it sit for at least 20 minutes. The more liquid removed from the tofu, the crispier the cooked tofu will be.

PER SERVING: Calories: 255; Fat: 11g; Total Carbohydrates: 29g; Net Carbs: 26g; Fiber: 3g; Protein: 15g; Sodium: 1161mg

TOFU SLICES WITH SRIRACHA MAYO

Serves 4 · Prep time: 15 minutes, plus 20 minutes pressing time /
Cook time: 20 minutes

NUT-FREE, VEGETARIAN

The perks of making your own crunchy tofu nuggets is that you can add different spices to the bread crumb mixture to change up the flavor.

1 (14-ounce) package extra-firm tofu, drained and pressed for 20 minutes

1 large egg

⅔ cup bread crumbs

1 tablespoon dried oregano

1 teaspoon chili powder

¼ teaspoon freshly ground black pepper

¼ teaspoon sea salt

½ cup low-fat mayonnaise

½ tablespoon sriracha

6 cups mixed greens

1. Cut the tofu into 16 equal slices and place on a plate. Set aside.

2. Preheat the oven to 400° F. Line a baking sheet with parchment paper.

3. In a shallow bowl, beat the egg. In another large bowl, mix the bread crumbs, oregano, chili powder, pepper, and salt.

4. Dip 1 slice of tofu in the egg, dredge it in the bread crumb mixture, and place it on the prepared baking sheet. Repeat with the rest of the tofu slices.

5. Bake for 20 minutes, or until golden brown, flipping the slices over after 10 minutes.

6. In a small bowl, mix the mayonnaise and sriracha.

7. Divide the mixed greens equally between 4 bowls and pair with the tofu slices. Divide the sauce into 4 small bowls and serve on the side for dipping.

> **SUBSTITUTION TIP:** If you don't eat eggs, mix 1 tablespoon flaxseed meal and 2½ tablespoons of water instead of using a beaten egg. Let the mixture sit for about 5 minutes before using.

PER SERVING (4 STRIPS): Calories: 257; Fat: 13g; Total Carbohydrates: 22g; Net Carbs: 19g; Fiber: 3g; Protein: 15g; Sodium: 327g

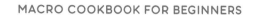

EASY TOFU PAD THAI

Serves 4 · Prep time: 10 minutes, plus 20 minutes pressing time /
Cook time: 20 minutes

DAIRY-FREE, VEGAN

Who needs to order takeout when you make this simple tofu pad thai yourself?

1 (14-ounce) package
   extra-firm tofu, drained
8 ounces pad thai brown
   rice noodles
2 tablespoons olive
   oil, divided
1½ teaspoons
   minced garlic
2 cups broccoli florets
2 scallions, green parts
   only, thinly sliced
2 tablespoons cornstarch
2 tablespoons creamy
   100% all-natural
   peanut butter
2 tablespoons low-sodium
   soy sauce
1 teaspoon sriracha

1. To press the tofu, wrap in 3 layers of paper towel and place between 2 plates. Place a weight on top and let it sit for at least 20 minutes. Cut the tofu into ½-inch cubes. Set aside.

2. Cook the pad thai noodles according to the package instructions.

3. Heat 1 tablespoon of olive oil in a nonstick skillet over medium heat. Add the garlic and sauté until slightly browned, about 30 seconds. Add the broccoli and sauté until some florets are lightly browned, 4 to 5 minutes. Add the scallions and mix well. Transfer to a bowl and set aside.

4. In a large bowl, toss the tofu with ½ tablespoon of olive oil. Add the cornstarch and stir until evenly coated.

5. Heat the remaining ½ tablespoon of olive oil in the skillet over medium-high heat. Add the tofu and cook, flipping the tofu every 2 to 3 minutes, until browned on all sides, 8 to 10 total minutes. Remove from the heat.

6. In a small bowl, mix the peanut butter, soy sauce, and sriracha. Pour the mixture over the tofu and mix well. Add the pad thai noodles and the broccoli and scallion mixture and toss together until combined. Serve immediately.

PER SERVING: Calories: 444; Fat: 17g; Total Carbohydrates: 57g; Net Carbs: 54g; Fiber: 3g; Protein: 17g; Sodium: 421mg

SWEET CRISPY TOFU BOWL

Serves 4 · Prep time: 10 minutes, plus 20 minutes tofu pressing time /
Cook time: 30 minutes

DAIRY-FREE, NUT-FREE, VEGAN

To get the tofu for these bowls nice and crispy, it's important to remove as much water as possible before cooking, which is why it should be pressed.

1 (14-ounce) package
   extra-firm tofu, drained
1½ cups quick brown rice
2 cups frozen
   shelled edamame
2 tablespoons low-sodium
   soy sauce
2 tablespoons
   reduced-sugar ketchup
2 teaspoons sriracha
1 tablespoon olive
   oil, divided
2 tablespoons cornstarch
1 small cucumber,
   thinly sliced
1 cup mango chunks

1. To press the tofu, wrap it in several layers of paper towel and place it between 2 plates. Place a weight on top and let it sit for at least 20 minutes. Cut the tofu into ½-inch cubes.

2. Cook the rice according to the package instructions.

3. In a medium pot, combine the edamame and enough water to cover and bring to a boil over medium-high heat. Cook until tender, 3 to 5 minutes. In a small bowl, mix the soy sauce, ketchup, and sriracha. Set aside.

4. In a large bowl, toss the tofu with ½ tablespoon of olive oil. Add the cornstarch and toss until evenly coated.

5. Heat the remaining ½ tablespoon of olive oil in a large nonstick skillet over medium-high heat. Add the tofu and cook, flipping the tofu over every 2 to 3 minutes, until all sides are equally crisp, about 8 to 10 minutes. Remove the pan from the heat and pour the soy sauce mixture over the tofu and mix well. Set aside.

6. Divide the rice equally between 4 bowls. Top with the edamame, cucumber, mango, and tofu mixture and serve immediately.

PER SERVING: Calories: 529; Fat: 15g; Total Carbohydrates: 77g; Net Carbs: 69g; Fiber: 8g; Protein: 25g; Sodium: 292mg

SESAME-EGG QUINOA BOWL

Serves 4 · Prep time: 10 minutes / Cook time: 35 minutes

DAIRY-FREE, VEGETARIAN

I like to include sesame seeds in meals as often as I can, because they contain nutrients like iron. The combination of the sesame seeds and hemp hearts provides a nutty flavor and a little extra crunch.

1 cup quinoa

1 tablespoon olive oil

½ large white onion, finely chopped

1 garlic clove, minced

2 large carrots, peeled and diced

1 green bell pepper, seeded and diced

2 large eggs, beaten

2 tablespoons low-sodium soy sauce

1 tablespoon sesame seeds

½ tablespoon hemp hearts

¼ teaspoon chili flakes

1. Cook the quinoa according to the package instructions. Set aside.

2. Heat the olive oil in a large nonstick skillet over medium heat. Add the onion and garlic and sauté for 1 minute. Add the carrots and bell pepper and cook until tender, 8 to 10 minutes. Reduce the heat to medium-low, push the vegetables to one side of the skillet, and add the eggs. Cook, using a spatula to move the eggs around as they cook until they are scrambled. Remove the pan from the heat.

3. Add the quinoa, soy sauce, sesame seeds, and hemp hearts and mix until combined. Divide the mixture equally between 4 bowls, top with the chili flakes, and serve.

> **SUBSTITUTION TIP:** To make this meal gluten-free, use gluten-free soy sauce (make sure to check the labels to ensure the soy sauce is processed in a completely gluten-free facility before buying it). To increase the protein, add more eggs or cooked chicken breast.

PER SERVING: Calories: 264; Fat: 9g; Total Carbohydrates: 35g; Net Carbs: 30g; Fiber: 5g; Protein: 11g; Sodium: 316mg

BAKED HALLOUMI AND VEGGIE SKEWERS

Serves 4 · Prep time: 10 minutes, plus 30 minutes skewer soaking time /
Cook time: 10 minutes

GLUTEN-FREE, NUT-FREE, VEGETARIAN

Halloumi is a semihard cheese, and like other cheeses delivers protein. One of the great things about this type of cheese is that it doesn't lose its shape when it's grilled or fried. If you're looking to add more protein to this meal, pair it with lean chicken or tofu skewers. This cooks up quickly, so it's a great choice if you're short on time.

Nonstick cooking spray

8 ounces Halloumi, cut into ½-inch cubes

1 green bell pepper, seeded and cut into 1-inch pieces

1 small zucchini, cut into ¾-inch slices

10 cherry tomatoes, halved

4 white button mushrooms

1 tablespoon olive oil

1 tablespoon dried oregano

1 tablespoon freshly squeezed lemon juice

1 teaspoon garlic powder

¼ teaspoon sea salt

1. Preheat the oven to 450°F. Lightly spray a large baking sheet with nonstick cooking spray. Soak wooden skewers in warm water for 30 minutes.

2. In a large bowl, mix the Halloumi, bell pepper, zucchini, cherry tomatoes, mushrooms, olive oil, oregano, lemon juice, garlic powder, and salt.

3. Thread the Halloumi and vegetables onto the wooden skewers. Place the skewers on the baking sheet and bake for 12 to 15 minutes, flipping the skewers after 8 minutes, or until the Halloumi is golden brown and the vegetables are slightly tender.

SUBSTITUTION TIP: Looking to change the flavor? Substitute 1 tablespoon of taco seasoning for the oregano and garlic powder. Pair it with baked tortilla chips, light sour cream, guacamole, and salsa to create Halloumi tacos on a stick.

PER SERVING: Calories: 227; Fat: 17g; Total Carbohydrates: 8g; Net Carbs: 6g; Fiber: 2g; Protein: 12g; Sodium: 549mg

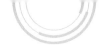

BLACK BEAN BURGER

Serves 4 · Prep time: 10 minutes / Cook time: 15 minutes
NUT-FREE, 30 MINUTES OR LESS, VEGETARIAN

Beans are loaded with nutrients—they're rich in protein and fiber—which makes them a great option for meatless meals. They contain an adequate amount of carbohydrates on their own, so I would suggest making the burger open face or leaving out the bun completely to control the carbohydrate content.

1 (15-ounce) can black
  beans, drained
  and rinsed
½ cup rolled oats
1 large egg white, beaten
⅓ cup shredded low-fat
  cheddar cheese
1½ tablespoons finely
  chopped white onion
1 tablespoon fajita
  seasoning
1 tablespoon chopped
  cilantro
Sea salt
Freshly ground
  black pepper
1 tablespoon olive oil
4 100% whole wheat buns
1 cup fresh baby spinach
1 cup fat-free sour cream

1. Pulse the black beans in a food processor until the beans are mashed. You may need to stop and scrape down the sides a few times. Transfer the beans to a large bowl.

2. Add the oats, egg white, cheese, onion, fajita seasoning, and cilantro to the beans and stir until combined. Season with salt and pepper. Form the mixture into 4 equal patties and place them on a plate.

3. Heat the olive oil in a large nonstick skillet over medium heat. Add the black bean patties and cook until heated through, about 3 minutes on each side.

4. Place the burgers on the whole wheat buns, top with spinach and dollops of sour cream, and serve.

> **SUBSTITUTION TIP:** To make this gluten-free, use gluten-free oats and a gluten-free bun or a lettuce wrap. Always read the labels to make sure that any seasonings are also gluten-free.

PER SERVING: Calories: 360; Fat: 9g; Total Carbohydrates: 53g; Net Carbs: 64g; Fiber: 9g; Protein: 17g; Sodium: 527mg

BLACK BEAN AND MUSHROOM QUESADILLAS

Serves 4 · Prep time: 10 minutes / Cook time: 15 minutes
NUT-FREE, 30 MINUTES OR LESS, VEGETARIAN

The Greek yogurt is a good protein alternative to mayonnaise and sour cream. In this recipe, it's used as a base for the sriracha lime dip.

1 (15-ounce) can black
   beans, including
   the liquid
1 teaspoon ground cumin
1 teaspoon garlic powder
Sea salt
Freshly ground
   black pepper
1½ cups plain nonfat
   Greek yogurt
2 tablespoons lime juice
1 tablespoon sriracha
½ tablespoon olive oil
1½ cups sliced white
   button mushrooms
2 cups fresh baby spinach
4 scallions, green parts
   only, thinly sliced
4 (10-inch) 100% whole
   wheat tortillas
Nonstick cooking spray
½ cup shredded
   reduced-fat mozzarella
   cheese, divided

1. In a small saucepan over medium-low heat, cook the black beans until heated through, about 5 minutes. Drain the beans and transfer to a bowl. Add the cumin and garlic powder and stir until combined. Taste, and season with the salt and pepper.

2. In a large bowl, mix the Greek yogurt, lime juice, and sriracha. Set aside.

3. Heat the olive oil in large skillet over medium-high heat. Add the mushrooms and cook for about 2 minutes. Stir in the spinach and scallions and cook until the spinach starts to wilt, about 1 minute. Remove from the heat. Taste, and season with salt and pepper. Transfer the mixture to a bowl and wipe out the skillet with a paper towel.

4. Spray 1 side of a tortilla with nonstick cooking spray and flip it over. Spread ¼ of the black bean mixture, ¼ of the vegetables, and 2 tablespoons of mozzarella cheese on half of the tortilla and fold it over.

5. Cook the quesadilla in the skillet over medium heat until lightly crisp and the cheese has melted. Repeat with the remaining tortillas.

6. Serve with the Greek yogurt sauce on the side.

PER SERVING: Calories: 408; Fat: 7g; Total Carbohydrates: 60g; Net Carbs: 51g; Fiber: 9g; Protein: 27g; Sodium: 668mg

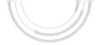

MEDITERRANEAN PINE NUT PENNE

Serves 4 · Prep time: 5 minutes / Cook time: 15 minutes

30 MINUTES OR LESS, VEGETARIAN

You're running late and realize you haven't prepared dinner. You're looking for a simple vegetarian meal that will keep you feeling full and still fit your macros for the day. You'll definitely want to bookmark this recipe. Add a chopped cooked chicken breast, canned tuna, or an egg to boost the protein.

8 ounces whole
  wheat penne

½ cup pine nuts, toasted

4 cups shredded spinach

½ cup crumbled
  reduced-fat feta cheese

½ cup black
  olives, drained

⅓ cup chopped sun-dried
  tomatoes

½ tablespoon
  hemp hearts

¼ teaspoon sea salt

¼ teaspoon freshly
  ground black pepper

1. Cook the penne according to the package instructions.

2. Toast the pine nuts in a small nonstick skillet over medium heat until golden brown and fragrant, 2 to 3 minutes. Transfer to a large bowl.

3. Add the spinach, feta, olives, sun-dried tomatoes, hemp hearts, salt, and pepper to the pine nuts and mix well.

4. Divide the penne between 4 bowls and top with equal amounts of the spinach mixture.

> **INGREDIENT TIP:** Pine nuts are a great source of polyunsaturated fats and contain many micronutrients, including iron, magnesium, and zinc.

PER SERVING: Calories: 396; Fat: 18g; Total Carbohydrates: 50g; Net Carbs: 43g; Fiber: 7g; Protein: 15g; Sodium: 452mg

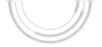

SPICY RICOTTA CHEESE LASAGNA

Serves 6 · Prep time: 10 minutes / Cook time: 35 to 40 minutes

NUT-FREE, VEGETARIAN

Choosing reduced-fat ricotta cheese when possible will help keep your overall calorie intake lower while supporting your macronutrient ratio and protein goals.

Nonstick cooking spray

6 whole wheat lasagna noodles

3 cups reduced-fat ricotta cheese

¾ tablespoon dried oregano

1 teaspoon chili powder

½ teaspoon olive oil

2 tablespoons minced white onion

1 garlic clove, minced

1 medium zucchini, finely diced

3 cups fresh baby spinach

2 cups low-sodium pasta sauce

½ cup shredded reduced-fat mozzarella cheese

1. Preheat the oven to 350° F. Lightly spray a lasagna baking dish with nonstick cooking spray.

2. Cook the lasagna noodles according to the package instructions. Drain and set aside.

3. In a medium bowl, mix the ricotta cheese, oregano, and chili powder. Set aside.

4. Heat the olive oil in a large nonstick skillet over medium heat. Add the onion and sauté until tender, 3 to 5 minutes. Add the garlic and sauté until the garlic starts to brown, about 30 seconds. Add the zucchini and cook until tender, 2 to 3 minutes. Add the spinach and stir until it begins to wilt. Remove from the heat and let sit until the spinach is completely wilted.

5. To assemble the lasagna: Spread out a thin layer of sauce in the baking pan and top with 3 lasagna noodles. Top with the ricotta mixture, the vegetable mixture, ½ of the remaining sauce, the remaining 3 lasagna noodles, and the remaining sauce. Sprinkle the mozzarella cheese over the top. Cover the baking pan with aluminum foil and use a fork to poke a few holes in the foil.

6. Bake for 20 to 25 minutes, or until the cheese has melted. Cut the lasagna into 6 equal portions and serve.

PER SERVING: Calories: 643; Fat: 19g; Total Carbohydrates: 84g; Net Carbs: 74g; Fiber: 10g; Protein: 40g; Sodium: 334mg

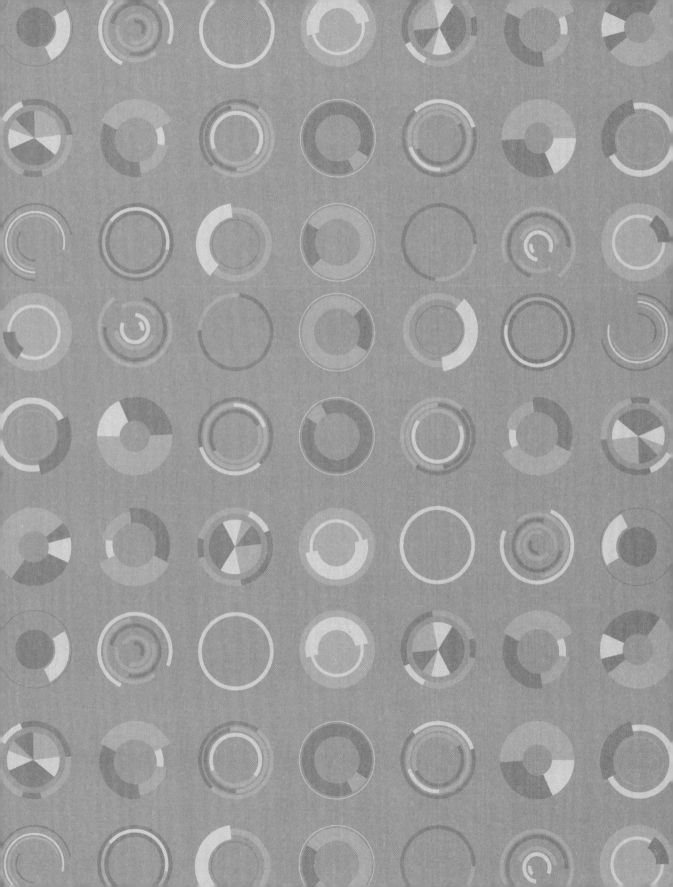

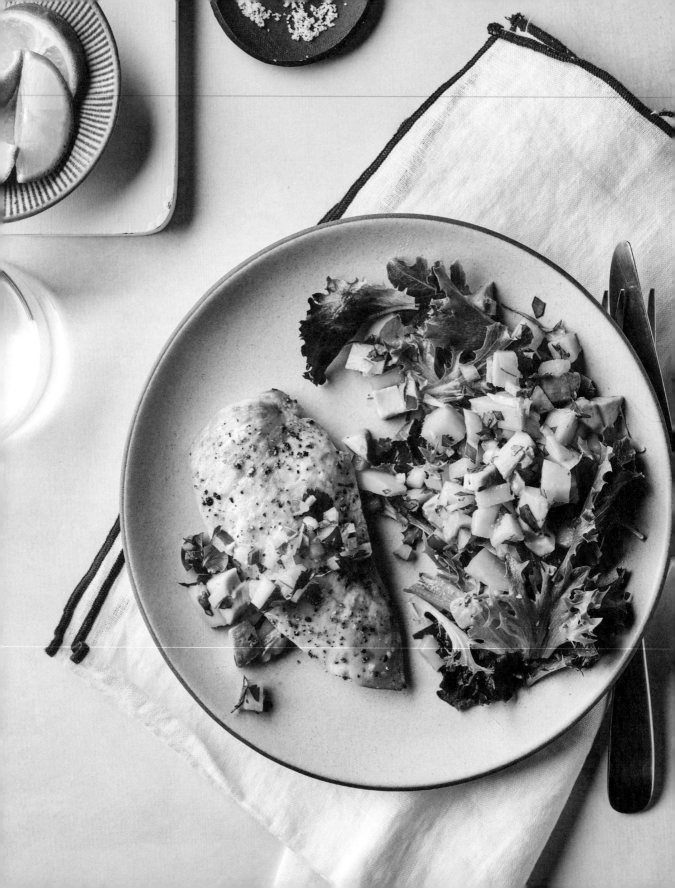

BASIL-CHICKEN PASTA

Serves 4 · Prep time: 15 minutes / Cook time: 25 minutes

Herbs and spices are a great way to add boosts of flavor to meals without packing in the sugar, fat, or calories. Although fresh herbs can have more flavor than their dried counterparts, dried can be more cost-efficient and convenient.

8 ounces whole wheat penne

1½ tablespoons olive oil, divided

12 ounces boneless, skinless chicken breast, cut into slices

1 teaspoon dried basil

3 garlic cloves, crushed

½ red bell pepper, seeded and chopped

1 green bell pepper, seeded and chopped

3 tablespoons Cashew Pesto (page 89)

1 cup fresh baby spinach

2 Roma tomatoes, chopped

½ cup shredded smoked low-fat cheddar cheese

1. Cook the pasta according to the package instructions. Drain and reserve ½ cup of the cooking water.

2. Heat 1 tablespoon of olive oil in large nonstick skillet over medium-high heat. Add the chicken and cook for 5 to 6 minutes. Flip over the chicken and cook until golden brown and cooked through, 4 to 6 minutes. Transfer to a plate and set aside.

3. In the same skillet, heat the remaining ½ tablespoon of oil over medium heat. Add the basil and cook, stirring, for 30 seconds. Add the garlic and cook, stirring, until lightly browned, about 30 seconds. Add the red and green bell peppers and the reserved pasta water and cook, stirring frequently, until the peppers are slightly tender, 4 to 5 minutes.

4. Add the pesto and cook, stirring, for 1 minute. Add the chicken, pasta, spinach, and tomatoes and mix well until combined. Remove the pan from the heat, sprinkle evenly with the cheese, and mix well.

5. Divide the mixture between 4 bowls and serve immediately.

> **SUBSTITUTION TIP:** If you don't have fresh garlic on hand, substitute ½ teaspoon of garlic powder.

PER SERVING: Calories: 481; Fat: 18g; Total Carbohydrates: 49g; Net Carbs: 42g; Fiber: 7g; Protein: 34g; Sodium: 272mg

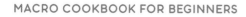

BALSAMIC CHICKEN AND VEGGIE SKEWERS

Serves 4 · Prep time: 10 minutes, plus 30 minutes marinating /
Cook time: 50 minutes

DAIRY-FREE, GLUTEN-FREE, NUT-FREE

You can use a variety of protein sources for skewers to fit your needs.

1½ cups quick brown rice

2 tablespoons bal-
  samic vinegar

2 tablespoons olive oil

⅛ teaspoon Dijon mustard

Sea salt

Freshly ground
  black pepper

1 pound boneless, skin-
  less chicken breast, cut
  into 1-inch pieces

1 medium zucchini, cut
  into 1-inch slices

1 yellow bell pepper,
  seeded and cut into
  1-inch pieces

1 large white onion, peeled
  and cut into 16 wedges

1. Cook the rice according to the package instructions.

2. Soak 12 wooden skewers in warm water for 30 minutes.

3. In a large zip-top plastic bag, mix the balsamic vinegar, olive oil, mustard, salt, and pepper. Add the chicken and seal the bag, making sure to remove as much air as possible. Squish the chicken around in the bag to ensure that all the pieces are evenly coated. Refrigerate for at least 30 minutes.

4. Preheat the oven to 450° F. Line 2 baking sheets with aluminum foil.

5. Remove the chicken from the marinade and discard the marinade. Thread the chicken, zucchini, bell pepper, and onion on the skewers.

6. Place skewers on the prepared baking sheets and bake for 25 to 30 minutes, flipping the skewers after 15 minutes, or until cooked through.

7. Divide the rice between 4 plates and top with skewers of meat and vegetables.

PREP TIP: Thickness of the chicken pieces can impact cooking time, so cut them all the same size.

PER SERVING: Calories: 497; Fat: 12g; Total Carbohydrates: 63g; Net Carbs: 59g; Fiber: 4g; Protein: 32g; Sodium: 64mg

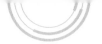

TURKEY MEATBALLS AND ZOODLES

Serves 2 · Prep time: 10 minutes / Cook time: 25 minutes
NUT–FREE

9 ounces extra-lean
    ground turkey

1 large egg, beaten

1½ tablespoons
    bread crumbs

½ tablespoon
    dried oregano

½ tablespoon Italian
    seasoning

1 teaspoon garlic powder

Sea salt

Freshly ground
    black pepper

⅓ cup grated reduced-fat
    Parmesan cheese

3 medium zucchini,
    ends trimmed

1 tablespoon olive oil

1 cup low-sodium mari-
    nara sauce

1. Preheat the oven to 375° F. Line a baking sheet with parchment paper.

2. In a large bowl, mix the turkey, egg, bread crumbs, oregano, Italian seasoning, and garlic powder. Season with the salt and pepper. Using your hands, form 8 equal balls. Using your finger, create a hole in the center of each ball. Press about 1½ tablespoons of cheese into the hole and pinch the meat together to enclose the cheese completely. Place the meatballs on the prepared baking sheet and bake for 25 to 28 minutes, or until center's internal temperature is 165° F.

3. While the meatballs are baking, use a spiralizer or vegetable peeler to make noodles or ribbons from the zucchini. Pat the zucchini noodles dry to remove excess water.

4. When the meatballs are nearly cooked, heat the oil in a nonstick skillet over medium heat. Add the zucchini noodles and sauté until they are slightly soft, 3 to 4 minutes. Be careful not to overcook–they can become soggy. Transfer the noodles to a plate.

5. In the same skillet over medium heat, combine the marinara sauce and meatballs and cook until warmed through.

6. To serve, divide the noodles between 2 plates and top with the meatballs and sauce. Season with the salt and pepper, to taste.

PER SERVING: Calories: 439; Fat: 25g; Total Carbohydrates: 22g; Net Carbs: 16g; Fiber: 6g; Protein: 36g; Sodium: 451mg

GARLIC-CHICKEN BURGER

To better suit your macronutrient needs, adjust the amount of ground chicken. Choose extra-lean poultry to limit the fat content. To increase the healthy fat, use more oil when cooking or add slices of avocado.

1 pound extra-lean
   ground chicken

1 large egg

¼ small white onion, diced

1 garlic clove, minced

1 tablespoon chopped
   fresh cilantro

1 tablespoon Worcester-
   shire sauce

1 tablespoon olive oil

½ cup shred-
   ded reduced-fat
   cheddar cheese

4 whole-grain buns

4 tomatoes, thickly sliced

1 cup fresh baby spinach

1. In a large bowl, mix the chicken, egg, onion, garlic, cilantro, and Worcestershire sauce. Form the mixture into 4 equal patties and place on a plate.

2. Heat the olive oil in a nonstick skillet over medium-high heat. Cook the patties in the skillet for 5 to 6 minutes. Flip the patties over and cook for 4 minutes. Sprinkle them with the cheese, cover, and cook until the patties are cooked through, 1 to 2 more minutes. Transfer the burgers to a plate and set aside.

3. Add the buns, cut-side down, to the skillet and cook until lightly browned, 3 minutes.

4. To serve, place a burger on each bun and top with the slices of tomatoes and the spinach.

LEFTOVER TIP: Reheat in a microwave oven, conventional oven, or on the stovetop to an internal temperature of 165° F.

PER SERVING: Calories: 378; Fat: 18g; Total Carbohydrates: 26g; Net Carbs: 23g; Fiber: 3g; Protein: 30g; Sodium: 460mg

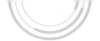

CUCUMBER-CHICKEN WRAPS

Serves 2 · Prep time: 10 minutes / Cook time: 15 minutes
30 MINUTES OR LESS

Hemp hearts are a protein-rich, plant-based food. You can easily incorporate them into your diet by consuming them raw or cooked. Since they don't contain gluten, they are a good substitute for wheat.

⅔ cups plain nonfat
  Greek yogurt

¼ cup shredded
  cucumber

2 garlic cloves, finely
  minced, divided

1 tablespoon hemp hearts

½ tablespoon freshly
  squeezed lemon juice

Sea salt

Freshly ground
  black pepper

½ tablespoon olive oil

6 ounces boneless, skin-
  less chicken breast, cut
  into thin slices

1½ teaspoons
  dried oregano

2 (10-inch) 100% whole
  wheat wraps

2 cups mixed greens

2 tablespoons crumbled
  reduced-fat feta cheese

1. In a medium bowl, mix the Greek yogurt, cucumber, half the garlic, the hemp hearts, and the lemon juice. Season with salt and pepper to taste. Set aside.

2. Heat the olive oil in a large nonstick skillet over medium-high heat. Add the remaining half of the garlic and sauté for 1 minute. Add the chicken and cook, stirring frequently, until golden brown and cooked through, 8 to 12 minutes. Add the oregano and season with salt and pepper to taste.

3. To assemble the wraps: Spread each wrap with the cucumber yogurt and top with the mixed greens, chicken, and feta. Wrap up and enjoy.

> **LEFTOVER TIP:** Store the dip and chicken separately in airtight containers for up to 3 days to reduce sogginess. Reheat the chicken in the microwave to an internal temperature of 165° F.

PER SERVING: Calories: 434; Fat: 12g; Total Carbohydrates: 44g; Net Carbs: 41g; Fiber: 3g; Protein: 36g; Sodium: 669mg

MAPLE-GINGER CHICKEN STIR-FRY

Serves 2 · Prep time: 1O minutes / Cook time: 4O minutes
DAIRY-FREE, NUT-FREE

Stir-fries are perfect for mixing your favorite protein combinations like chicken and egg or tofu and nuts.

¾ cup quick brown rice

3 tablespoons low-sodium soy sauce

2 tablespoons maple syrup

3 tablespoons water

1 tablespoon olive oil, divided

2 large carrots, peeled and diced

1 green bell pepper, seeded and diced

1½ teaspoons minced garlic

1 teaspoon minced ginger

10 ounces boneless, skinless chicken breast, cut into 1-inch pieces

Sea salt

Freshly ground black pepper

1. Cook the rice according to the package instructions.

2. In a small bowl, mix soy sauce, maple syrup, and water. Set aside.

3. Heat ½ tablespoon of olive oil in a large nonstick skillet over medium heat. Add the carrots and cook, stirring, for 4 to 5 minutes. Add the bell pepper to cook until the carrots are tender and slightly soft, 3 to 5 minutes. Transfer the mixture to a bowl.

4. In the same skillet, heat the remaining ½ tablespoon of oil over medium-high heat. Add the garlic and ginger and sauté for 1 minute. Add the chicken and cook, stirring frequently, until golden brown and cooked through, 8 to 12 minutes. Reduce the heat, add the vegetable mixture and the sauce, and mix well. Season with salt and pepper to taste.

5. Divide the recipe between 2 bowls and top with the chicken and vegetable mixture. Serve immediately.

LEFTOVER TIP: Refrigerate in an airtight container for up to 3 days. Reheat in a microwave oven, conventional oven, or on the stovetop to an internal temperature of 165° F.

PER SERVING: Calories: 597; Fat: 13g; Total Carbohydrates: 79g; Net Carbs: 73g; Fiber: 6g; Protein: 41g; Sodium: 887mg

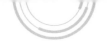

CASHEW AND FETA STUFFED CHICKEN

Serves 4 · Prep time: 15 minutes / Cook time: 30 minutes
GLUTEN-FREE

Stuffed chicken breasts are pretty filling, so I usually pair them with a simple side salad, which makes a very satisfying meal. If you're looking to make this a larger meal, consider serving the chicken with orzo and roasted vegetables instead.

3 teaspoons olive
  oil, divided
⅓ cup finely chopped
  scallions
2 garlic cloves, minced
3 cups finely
  chopped spinach
¾ cup crumbled
  reduced-fat feta cheese
2 tablespoons
  crushed cashews
2 tablespoons minced
  fresh parsley
¼ teaspoon chili powder
½ teaspoon sea
  salt, divided
4 (4-ounce) boneless,
  skinless chicken breasts

1. Preheat the oven to 350° F. Line a baking sheet with aluminum foil.

2. Heat 1 teaspoon of olive oil in a large nonstick skillet over medium heat. Add the scallions and garlic and sauté for 1 minute. Add the spinach and cook, stirring, until it starts to wilt, 1 to 2 minutes. Remove from the heat. Add the feta, cashews, parsley, chili powder, and ¼ teaspoon of salt. Set aside.

3. Cut a 2-inch pocket in the center of each chicken breast and divide the spinach mixture between the 4 chicken breasts.

4. Using a basting brush, spread the remaining 2 teaspoons of olive oil over the chicken. Season with the remaining ¼ teaspoon of salt and pepper. Bake stuffed breasts on the prepared baking sheet for 25 to 30 minutes, or until the chicken is no longer pink and the juices run clear. Serve immediately.

PREP TIP: If the filling in the chicken breast is spilling out of the pocket, secure with 1 or 2 wooden toothpicks. Soak the toothpicks in water for at least 20 minutes to prevent burning in the oven. Remove the toothpicks prior to serving.

PER SERVING: Calories: 275; Fat: 14g; Total Carbohydrates: 4g; Net Carbs: 3g; Fiber: 1g; Protein: 31g; Sodium: 567mg

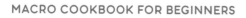

CHICKEN WITH MANGO SALSA

Serves 4 · Prep time: 10 minutes / Cook time: 25 minutes
DAIRY-FREE, GLUTEN-FREE, NUT-FREE

Mangos have a natural sweetness that adds a lot of flavor without too much added sugar. Although mangos are not always in season, they are available frozen in most supermarkets, and will work just as well in this recipe.

1 tablespoon olive oil

4 (4-ounce) boneless, skinless chicken breasts

½ teaspoon sea salt

¼ teaspoon freshly ground black pepper

1 avocado, pitted, peeled, and diced

1 cup diced fresh or frozen mango

1 garlic clove, minced

¼ cup minced red onion

¼ cup chopped fresh cilantro

2 tablespoons lime juice

1 teaspoon olive oil

8 cups mixed greens

1. Preheat the oven to 400° F. Line a baking sheet with aluminum foil.

2. Using a basting brush, spread the olive oil over the chicken and season with the salt and pepper. Arrange the chicken on the prepared baking sheet and bake for 20 to 25 minutes, or until cooked through.

3. While the chicken bakes, in a large bowl, mix the avocado, mango, garlic, red onion, and cilantro. Add the lime juice and oil and stir until combined. Cover with plastic wrap and refrigerate until ready to serve.

4. Place a chicken breast on each of 4 plates. Divide the mixed greens between the plates and top with mango salsa.

> **LEFTOVER TIP:** Refrigerate the mango salsa and chicken in separate airtight containers for up to 3 days. Reheat in a microwave oven.

PER SERVING: Calories: 313; Fat: 16g; Total Carbohydrates: 16g; Net Carbs: 10g; Fiber: 6g; Protein: 29g; Sodium: 292mg

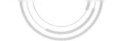

CHICKEN PARMESAN

Serves 4 · Prep time: 10 minutes / Cook time: 45 minutes
NUT-FREE

This recipe is loaded with protein from the chicken, egg, egg whites, and Parmesan and mozzarella cheeses. Try using lower-fat options for the cheeses.

1½ cups quinoa

Nonstick cooking spray

1 cup bread crumbs

1 tablespoon
   dried oregano

1 teaspoon
   smoked paprika

¼ cup grated reduced-fat
   Parmesan cheese

1 large egg

2 large egg whites

2 tablespoons
   all-purpose flour

4 (4½-ounce) bone-
   less, skinless chicken
   breasts, each halved
   lengthwise

1 cup low-sodium mari-
   nara sauce

¼ cup shredded
   reduced-fat mozza-
   rella cheese

8 cups mixed greens

1. Make the quinoa according to the package instructions.

2. Preheat the oven to 450° F. Lightly spray a baking sheet with nonstick cooking spray.

3. In a shallow dish, combine the bread crumbs, oregano, paprika, and Parmesan cheese. Set aside. In another shallow dish, beat together the egg and egg whites. Set aside.

4. Sprinkle the flour over the chicken breasts, making sure both sides are lightly coated.

5. Using one hand, dip a chicken breast in the egg mixture; using the other hand, press the egg-coated chicken breast into the bread crumb mixture. Place the chicken on the baking sheet. Repeat with the remaining chicken. Sprinkle any remaining bread crumb mixture over the chicken breasts.

6. Bake for 25 minutes. Pour ¼ cup of marinara sauce over each chicken breast and top each with 1 tablespoon of mozzarella cheese. Bake for 3 to 5 minutes more, or until the cheese is melted.

7. Divide the quinoa among 4 bowls. Top with the greens and the chicken. Serve hot.

PER SERVING: Calories: 568; Fat: 12g; Total Carbohydrates: 65g; Net Carbs: 57g; Fiber: 8g; Protein: 49g; Sodium: 394mg

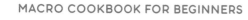

PESTO CHICKEN

Serves 4 · Prep time: 5 minutes / Cook time: 25 minutes
GLUTEN-FREE

Although this recipe is higher in protein and fat, it's a great dish to pair with pasta like linguine to increase the carbohydrate content. To complete the meal, pair it with a mixed green salad with a simple squeeze of lemon juice for the dressing.

1 pound boneless, skin-less chicken breasts

½ teaspoon sea salt

¼ teaspoon freshly ground black pepper

¼ cup reduced-fat French onion dip

¾ cup nonfat plain Greek yogurt

2 tablespoons olive oil

2 garlic cloves, minced

2 tablespoons Cashew Pesto (page 89)

1 cup halved cherry tomatoes

½ cup grated reduced-fat Parmesan cheese

⅛ cup thinly sliced fresh basil

1. Season the chicken with salt and pepper and set it aside on a plate.

2. In a small bowl, mix the French onion dip and Greek yogurt. Set aside.

3. Heat the olive oil in a nonstick skillet over medium-high heat. Add the garlic and cook for 1 minute. Add the chicken and cook for 5 to 6 minutes. Flip over the chicken and cook for 4 to 6 minutes. Add the pesto and continue to cook until browned and cooked through, another 1 to 2 minutes. Add the yogurt mixture and mix well. Increase the heat to high and bring to a boil.

4. Reduce the heat to medium, add the tomatoes, and cook until they soften, about 2 to 3 minutes. Reduce the heat to medium-low and simmer for 4 to 5 minutes. Top with the Parmesan cheese.

5. Place the chicken on a serving plate and garnish with the basil.

> **PREP TIP:** Although pesto is a great source of healthy fat, it is calorically dense. A small amount goes a long way, so be sure to measure out the exact portion needed. You can also use jarred pesto from the supermarket.

PER SERVING: Calories: 361; Fat: 20g; Total Carbohydrates: 11g; Net Carbs: 10g; Fiber: 1g; Protein: 34g; Sodium: 834mg

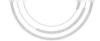

PINEAPPLE-SHRIMP BOWL

Serves 4 · Prep time: 10 minutes / Cook time: 30 minutes

DAIRY-FREE, GLUTEN-FREE

If you're looking for a protein source that is quick and easy to make, shrimp is a great option. It absorbs flavors easily and is often paired with pesto on pizza. Taking that same combo, this easy rice bowl meets your macronutrient ratio and can be made in 15 minutes.

1½ cups quick brown rice
½ tablespoon olive oil
1 garlic clove, minced
1½ cups baby shrimp
¼ teaspoon chili powder
2 cups fresh baby spinach
¼ cup pesto
½ cup pineapple chunks

1. Cook the rice according to the package instructions.

2. Heat the oil in a large nonstick skillet over medium-high heat. Add the garlic and sauté for 1 minute. Add the shrimp and cook until pink and cooked through, 4 to 6 minutes. Add the chili powder and spinach and cook, stirring, for 1 minute.

3. Reduce the heat to medium, add the pesto, and stir well until the shrimp is evenly coated. Remove from heat. Add the rice and stir until combined. Top with pineapple chunks and serve.

> **SUBSTITUTION TIP:** If fresh pineapples are not available, it's fine to use canned ones. Before adding the canned pineapples, drain and rinse them.

PER SERVING: Calories: 419; Fat: 13g; Total Carbohydrates: 58g; Net Carbs: 55g; Fiber: 3g; Protein: 17g; Sodium: 577mg

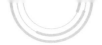

SUN-DRIED TOMATO AND PARMESAN SHRIMP PASTA

Serves 4 · Prep time: 10 minutes / Cook time: 15 minutes
NUT-FREE, 30 MINUTES OR LESS

Sun-dried tomatoes add a punch of flavor, and while they can be purchased packed in oil, choose the ones that are not, which will help make tracking macros easier. The oil can easily add up and impact your fat intake.

8 ounces whole wheat bow tie pasta, cooked

2 teaspoons olive oil, divided

1½ cups baby shrimp

¾ teaspoon garlic powder

¼ teaspoon chili flakes

6 cups fresh baby spinach

4 teaspoons all-purpose flour

1 cup 1% milk

2 tablespoons chopped sun-dried tomatoes

2 scallions, thinly sliced

½ cup grated reduced-fat Parmesan cheese

1. Cook the pasta according to the package instructions.

2. Heat 1½ teaspoons of olive oil in a large nonstick skillet over medium-high heat. Add the shrimp and cook until pink and cooked through, 4 to 6 minutes. Transfer to a plate.

3. In the same skillet, heat the remaining ½ teaspoon of olive oil over medium heat. Add the garlic powder and chili flakes and cook for 30 seconds. Add the spinach and cook, stirring, until it begins to wilt, 1 to 2 minutes.

4. In a small bowl, whisk together the flour and milk. Add the mixture to the skillet and cook, stirring constantly, until combined. Reduce the heat to low; add the shrimp, pasta, sun-dried tomatoes, and scallions to the skillet and mix well. Remove from heat, add the Parmesan cheese, and stir until combined. Serve immediately.

LEFTOVER TIP: Store in an airtight container in the refrigerator for up to 2 days. Adjust the pasta amount if you are trying to meet a specific carbohydrate amount for the meal or day for the day.

PER SERVING: Calories: 352; Fat: 7g; Total Carbohydrates: 51g; Net Carbs: 45g; Fiber: 6g; Protein: 25g; Sodium: 681mg

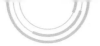

BAKED SALMON WITH GREEN BEANS

Serves 4 · Prep time: 10 minutes / Cook time: 30 minutes

DAIRY-FREE, GLUTEN-FREE, NUT-FREE

Salmon is great on two fronts, because it will increase your omega-3 intake while also providing protein. Pair it with various vegetables and grains. To adjust the carbohydrate intake, alter the amount of rice.

1½ cups quick brown rice

Nonstick cooking spray

1 (16-ounce) salmon fillet

2½ teaspoons olive oil, divided

¼ teaspoon sea salt

¼ teaspoon freshly ground black pepper, divided

4 cups green beans, trimmed

1 garlic clove, minced

½ teaspoon freshly squeezed lemon juice

1. Cook the rice according to the package instructions.

2. Preheat the oven to 450° F. Line 2 baking sheets with aluminum foil and lightly spray with nonstick cooking spray.

3. Place the salmon, skin-side down, on the prepared baking sheet. Using a basting brush, coat the salmon with 2 teaspoons of oil and season with the salt and ⅛ teaspoon of pepper.

4. In a large bowl, toss the green beans with the remaining ½ teaspoon of oil, garlic, lemon juice, and the remaining ⅛ teaspoon of pepper. Spread out the green beans on the other baking sheet. Bake both trays at the same time for 10 to 12 minutes, or until cooked through. Divide the salmon and green beans between 4 plates and serve with the rice.

> **COOKING TIP:** To add more flavor without greatly impacting the nutrient profile, add another garlic clove, add more salt and pepper, or increase the amount of lemon juice.

PER SERVING: Calories: 476; Fat: 12g; Total Carbohydrates: 61g; Net Carbs: 46g; Fiber: 5g; Protein: 30g; Sodium: 175mg

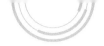

MAPLE SALMON WITH MINI POTATOES

Serves 4 · Prep time: 10 minutes / Cook time: 20 minutes
DAIRY-FREE, GLUTEN-FREE, NUT-FREE, 30 MINUTES OR LESS

Salmon is a great source of omega-3 fatty acids. And when you bake it along with mini potatoes on a sheet pan, it's a recipe that requires minimal cleanup.

3 tablespoons olive oil, divided

2 tablespoons maple syrup

1 tablespoon balsamic vinegar

1 tablespoon minced shallot

½ teaspoon sea salt, divided

¼ teaspoon freshly ground black pepper, divided

4 (3-ounce) salmon fillets, of similar thickness

24 ounces mini potatoes, each halved

6 cups mixed greens

Lemon juice

1. Preheat the oven to 450° F. Line 2 baking sheets with aluminum foil. In a medium bowl, mix 1 tablespoon of olive oil, the maple syrup, balsamic vinegar, shallot, ¼ teaspoon of salt, and ⅛ teaspoon of pepper. Set aside.

2. Place the salmon skin-side down on the prepared baking sheet. Using a basting brush, coat the salmon with the maple dressing.

3. In a large bowl, toss the mini potatoes with the remaining 2 tablespoons of olive oil, the remaining ¼ teaspoon of salt, and the remaining ⅛ teaspoon of pepper. Spread out the potatoes on the second baking sheet. Place both trays in the oven and bake 10 to 12 minutes, or until the salmon is cooked through. Drizzle any remaining dressing over the salmon and set aside. Continue to bake the mini potatoes for a total of 20 to 25 minutes, or until just tender.

4. Place a salmon fillet on each of 4 plates. Place 1½ cups of mixed greens on each plate and drizzle with lemon juice to taste.

> **COOKING TIP:** The thickness of the salmon can impact cooking time. To check for doneness, insert a fork into the thickest part of the salmon. The salmon should be opaque and flake easily. Continue to cook for a few minutes if not done.

PER SERVING: Calories: 386; Fat: 16g; Total Carbohydrates: 40g; Net Carbs: 35g; Fiber: 5g; Protein: 22g; Sodium: 345mg

LEMON-TUNA QUINOA BOWL

Serves 2 · Prep time: 5 minutes / Cook time: 30 minutes

GLUTEN-FREE

Simple meals can make tracking macros easier, especially when you are first learning how to hit your specific ratio. Canned tuna adds protein to a meal, though you should choose tuna canned in water to avoid any added fat and calories from oil-packed versions, which can impact the macronutrient ratio.

½ cup quinoa

1 (5-ounce) can light tuna packed in water, drained

3 scallions, green parts only, finely chopped

½ cup nonfat plain Greek yogurt

¼ cup crumbled reduced-fat feta cheese

3 tablespoons low-fat mayonnaise

2 tablespoons hemp hearts

½ tablespoon freshly squeezed lemon juice

4 cups mixed greens

½ cup halved cherry tomatoes

Sea salt

Freshly ground black pepper

1. Cook quinoa according to the package instructions.

2. In a large bowl, mix the tuna, scallions, Greek yogurt, feta, mayonnaise, hemp hearts, and lemon juice.

3. Assemble the bowls: Divide the mixed greens equally between 2 bowls. Top with the tuna mixture and the tomatoes. Season with salt and pepper to taste.

PREP TIP: To reduce cooking time, make enough quinoa for 2 meals and store in an airtight container in the refrigerator for up to 4 days.

PER SERVING: Calories: 188; Fat: 6g; Total Carbohydrates: 20g; Net Carbs: 17g; Fiber: 3g; Protein: 15g; Sodium: 194mg

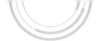

BAKED FISH AND CHIPS

Serves 4 · Prep time: 15 minutes / Cook time: 25 minutes
DAIRY-FREE

When you bake fish with olive oil, you can reduce the saturated fat usually found in fish and chips while increasing the healthy fat content. The inclusion of all-bran flakes and hemp hearts provide fiber.

Nonstick cooking spray

¼ cup all-bran flakes

2 pounds mini potatoes

1½ tablespoons olive oil

¾ teaspoon sea
salt, divided

½ teaspoon freshly
ground black
pepper, divided

¾ cup bread crumbs

1 tablespoon hemp hearts

½ tablespoon
dried parsley

½ teaspoon garlic powder

½ teaspoon chili powder

1 large egg, beaten

1 (16-ounce) halibut fillet,
cut into 4 pieces

1. Preheat the oven to 450° F. Line 2 baking sheets with aluminum foil and coat with nonstick cooking spray.

2. In a food processor, pulse the bran flakes until they have a flourlike consistency. Set aside.

3. Cut the mini potatoes in half lengthwise and place in a large bowl. Add olive oil, ½ teaspoon of sea salt, and ¼ teaspoon of pepper and stir until combined. Spread out the potatoes on the prepared baking sheet.

4. Bake for 10 minutes. Turn over the potatoes and continue to bake for 10 to 15 more minutes, or until just tender.

5. While potatoes are baking, in a shallow bowl, mix the bran flake flour, bread crumbs, hemp hearts, parsley, garlic powder, chili powder, the remaining ¼ teaspoon of salt, and the remaining ¼ teaspoon of pepper. In another shallow bowl, beat the egg.

6. Coat a piece of fish in the egg and then dredge in the bread crumb mixture. Place on the prepared baking sheet. Repeat with the rest of the fish.

7. Bake for 10 to 14 minutes or until the center of the fish is opaque. Serve hot with the mini potatoes.

PER SERVING: Calories: 523; Fat: 23g; Total Carbohydrates: 54g; Net Carbs: 48g; Fiber: 6g; Protein: 25g; Sodium: 618mg

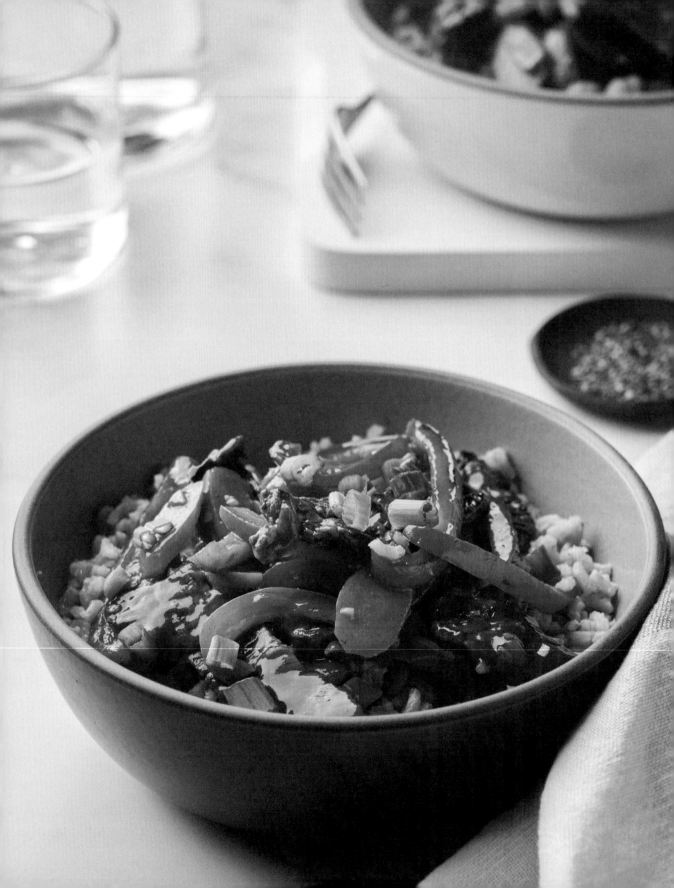

BEEF AND
PORK MAINS

MUSHROOM AND CHEDDAR CHEESEBURGERS

Serves 4 · Prep time: 10 minutes / Cook time: 15 minutes
30 MINUTES OR LESS

If you're looking to make a fast burger that can easily work within a macronutrient ratio, try this recipe. This recipe has them sandwiched in burger buns, but you can also try them open-faced or wrapped in lettuce leaves, a great option if you're trying to lower your carbs.

12 ounces extra-lean
  ground beef

1 large egg, beaten

½ cup shredded low-fat
  cheddar cheese

⅓ cup diced mushrooms

¼ cup finely chopped
  scallions

1 tablespoon chopped
  fresh cilantro

1 teaspoon Worcester-
  shire sauce

½ teaspoon sea salt

¼ teaspoon freshly
  ground black pepper

1 tablespoon olive oil

4 100% whole wheat
  burger buns

1. In a large bowl, mix the ground beef, egg, cheese, mushrooms, scallions, cilantro, Worcestershire sauce, salt, and pepper. Using your hands, shape the mixture into 4 equal patties.

2. Heat the olive oil in a large nonstick skillet over medium-high heat. Add the patties and cook until cooked through, 4 to 5 minutes on each side.

3. Place each patty on a bun and add your desired toppings.

> **COOKING TIP:** To avoid added sugars or too many calories, top your burgers with thick tomato slices, onions, lettuce, or pickles, all of which add a lot of flavor but not many calories.

PER SERVING: Calories: 321; Fat: 14g; Total Carbohydrates: 20g; Net Carbs: 18g; Fiber: 2g; Protein: 28g; Sodium: 629mg

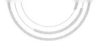

STEAK AND BELL PEPPER FAJITAS

Serves 4 · Prep time: 10 minutes / Cook time: 15 minutes
DAIRY-FREE, NUT-FREE, 30 MINUTES OR LESS

This is a wonderful midweek meal that goes from kitchen to table in under 30 minutes. Add more steak or pair the fajitas with a lime-Greek yogurt sauce to increase the protein content.

12 ounces top sirloin steak, cut into thin slices

2 teaspoons paprika

1 teaspoon ground cumin

½ teaspoon garlic powder

½ teaspoon freshly ground black pepper

½ teaspoon sea salt

1½ tablespoons olive oil, divided

1 red bell pepper, seeded and thinly sliced

1 green bell pepper, seeded and thinly sliced

1 medium white onion, thinly sliced

4 (8-inch) whole wheat tortillas

½ cup fresh salsa

1. In a large bowl, toss the steak with the paprika, cumin, garlic powder, pepper, and salt until evenly coated.

2. Heat 1 tablespoon of olive oil in a large nonstick skillet over medium-high heat. Add the steak and cook, stirring frequently, until browned, 8 to 10 minutes. Transfer to a plate and set aside.

3. In the same skillet, heat the remaining ½ tablespoon of oil over medium heat. Add the red and green bell peppers and cook, stirring frequently, until tender, 4 to 5 minutes. Add the onion and continue to cook until the onion is soft, 3 to 5 minutes. Add the steak to the skillet and stir until combined. Transfer the mixture to the plate and set aside.

4. Wipe out the skillet with paper towels. Warm up the tortillas in a skillet over medium-high heat.

5. Divide the fajita filling equally between the tortillas. Top with the salsa and serve.

> **COOKING TIP:** If the vegetables start to dry out while you're cooking the onion, lower the heat and add 1 to 2 tablespoons of water and continue to stir.

PER SERVING: Calories: 375; Fat: 19g; Total Carbohydrates: 28g; Net Carbs: 21g; Fiber: 7g; Protein: 23g; Sodium: 722mg

QUINOA, TOMATO, AND BEEF STUFFED PEPPERS

Serves 4 · Prep time: 10 minutes / Cook time: 45 minutes
GLUTEN-FREE, NUT-FREE

Bell peppers are packed with nutrients and fiber, and ground beef and quinoa contribute protein. They are also pretty enough to serve to guests.

½ cup quinoa

1 tablespoon olive oil

2 scallions, both green and white parts, finely chopped

3 garlic cloves, minced

8 ounces extra-lean ground beef

2 teaspoons minced fresh basil

½ teaspoon sea salt

¼ teaspoon freshly ground black pepper

½ cup reduced-sodium tomato sauce

4 red bell peppers, tops removed and seeded

½ cup shredded reduced-fat mozzarella cheese

1. Cook the quinoa according to the package instructions.

2. Preheat the oven to 350° F. Have a shallow baking dish ready.

3. Heat the olive oil in a large nonstick skillet over medium-high heat. Add the scallions and garlic and sauté for 1 minute. Add the ground beef and cook, breaking it apart using a wooden spoon, until it is browned and cooked through, 6 to 8 minutes.

4. Add the basil, salt, pepper, and tomato sauce and stir until combined. Remove from the heat, add the quinoa, and stir until combined.

5. Stand the peppers in the baking dish and stuff each one with equal amounts of beef and quinoa mixture. Cover the baking dish with aluminum foil and bake for 10 to 15 minutes, or until the peppers are tender. Sprinkle the cheese over the top and bake for an additional 5 minutes, or until the cheese is melted.

> **LEFTOVER TIP:** Tightly wrap each bell pepper in aluminum foil and refrigerate for up to 3 days. Reheat in the oven until heated through.

PER SERVING: Calories: 269; Fat: 10g; Total Carbohydrates: 24g; Net Carbs: 19g; Fiber: 5g; Protein: 20g; Sodium: 369mg

BEEF TACOS ON A STICK

Serves 4 • Prep time: 10 minutes, plus 1 hour marinating /
Cook time: 15 minutes

DAIRY-FREE, GLUTEN-FREE, NUT-FREE

This recipe is high in protein, but you can increase or decrease the beef to meet your macronutrient ratio. If you are trying to increase both fat and carbohydrate intake, pair this recipe with baked tortilla chips, lettuce, guacamole, and fresh salsa.

1 small white
  onion, chopped
Juice of 1 lime
1 teaspoon ground cumin
1 teaspoon chili powder
½ teaspoon garlic powder
¼ teaspoon sea salt
¼ teaspoon freshly
  ground black pepper
12 ounces beef sirloin tips,
  cut into 1-inch cubes
Nonstick cooking spray
1 red bell pepper,
  seeded and cut into
  1-inch pieces
1 large white onion, peeled
  and cut into 8 wedges

1. In a food processor, combine the onion, lime juice, cumin, chili powder, garlic powder, salt, and pepper and puree until smooth.

2. Transfer the mixture to a large zip-top plastic bag. Add the sirloin tips, seal, and use your hands to squish around the beef so it's evenly coated in the marinade. Refrigerate for at least 1 hour.

3. Preheat the broiler. Spray the broiler rack with nonstick cooking spray. Remove the beef from the plastic bag and discard the marinade. Thread the beef, pepper, and onion alternately onto 8 to 12 metal skewers.

4. Place the skewers on the broiler rack and broil for 5 minutes. Turn over the skewers and broil for another 4 to 5 minutes, or until the beef is cooked through.

> **PREP TIP:** If you are short on time, you can use 1½ teaspoons of prepackaged low-sodium taco seasoning instead of the spices in the recipe.

PER SERVING: Calories: 149; Fat: 4g; Total Carbohydrates: 9g; Net Carbs: 7g; Fiber: 2g; Protein: 19g; Sodium: 186mg

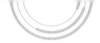

ROSEMARY AND THYME STEAK

Serves 4 · Prep time: 10 minutes / Cook time: 15 minutes
GLUTEN-FREE, NUT-FREE, 30 MINUTES OR LESS

If you're craving a steak that isn't calorically dense, you must try this recipe. To increase the carbohydrate content, pair the steak with baked potatoes or add a whole grain. It will be a classic and very satisfying dinner.

2½ tablespoons olive oil, divided

4 (4-ounce) top sirloin steaks, each 1 inch thick

½ teaspoon freshly ground black pepper, plus more as needed

½ teaspoon sea salt, plus more as needed

1 sprig fresh rosemary

1 sprig fresh thyme

2 garlic cloves, minced

1 tablespoon butter

1 pound green beans, trimmed

1. Heat 1½ tablespoons of olive oil in a large non-stick skillet over medium-high heat. Season the steaks with the pepper and salt. Add the rosemary, thyme, and garlic to the skillet. Add the steak and cook until browned, 3 to 4 minutes on each side.

2. Add the butter and continue to cook the steak, basting the steak with the butter constantly, for 1 to 2 minutes. Remove the skillet from the heat.

3. Bring a large pot of water to a boil over high heat. Add the green beans and cook until tender, 4 to 5 minutes.

4. Drain and toss the green beans with the remaining 1 tablespoon of olive oil and season with the salt and pepper to taste.

> **SUBSTITUTION TIP:** Although fresh thyme and rosemary offer more flavoring for this steak, you can use 1 teaspoon dried rosemary and 1 teaspoon of dried thyme instead.

PER SERVING: Calories: 352; Fat: 24g; Total Carbohydrates: 8g; Net Carbs: 5g; Fiber: 3g; Protein: 26g; Sodium: 323mg

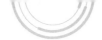

ORANGE–GINGER BEEF

Serves 4 · Prep time: 15 minutes / Cook time: 30 minutes
DAIRY-FREE, NUT-FREE

If you don't have freshly squeezed orange juice for this recipe, store-bought orange juice with no pulp can also be used.

1½ cups quick brown rice

⅓ cup freshly squeezed orange juice, no pulp

4 garlic cloves, minced, divided

1 teaspoon minced ginger

2 tablespoons low-sodium soy sauce

1 teaspoon cornstarch

2 teaspoons water

2 tablespoons olive oil, divided

12 ounces top sirloin steak, thinly sliced

1 cup sliced carrots cut into ¼-inch pieces

1 red bell pepper, seeded and thinly sliced

1 green bell pepper, seeded and thinly sliced

Sea salt

Freshly ground black pepper

1. Cook the rice according to the package instructions. Set aside.

2. To make the marinade, in a small saucepan, combine the orange juice, half the garlic, the ginger, and the soy sauce, and bring it to a boil over medium-high heat.

3. In a small bowl, mix the cornstarch and water. Add the mixture to the saucepan, lower the heat to low, and stir until combined. Cook, stirring occasionally, until the marinade thickens, 6 to 8 minutes. Set aside.

4. Heat 1 tablespoon of the oil in a large nonstick skillet over medium-high heat. Add the steak and cook, stirring frequently, until browned, 5 to 8 minutes. Transfer to a plate.

5. In the same skillet, heat the remaining 1 tablespoon of oil. Add the remaining garlic and sauté for 1 minute. Add the carrots and cook for 4 to 5 minutes. Add the red and green bell peppers and cook until tender, 4 to 6 minutes.

6. Add the steak and the sauce and mix well.

7. Divide the rice between 4 plates. Top with the steak, including the sauce. Add salt and pepper to taste and serve.

PER SERVING: Calories: 528; Fat: 18g; Total Carbohydrates: 65g; Net Carbs: 60g; Fiber: 5g; Protein: 25g; Sodium: 329mg

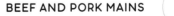

TOMATO BEEF AND BEAN CHILI

Serves 6 · Prep time: 10 minutes / Cook time: 35 minutes
DAIRY-FREE, GLUTEN-FREE, NUT-FREE

This hearty, protein-packed meal is the perfect option for a cold, blustery day. The beans not only provide protein but are also packed with fiber—both of which can help make you feel fuller longer.

1 tablespoon olive oil

½ large white onion, chopped

3 garlic cloves, minced

1 tablespoon tomato paste

1 pound extra-lean ground beef

1½ tablespoons chili powder

1 teaspoon ground cumin

1 teaspoon dried oregano

½ teaspoon paprika

Sea salt

Freshly ground black pepper

1 (15-ounce) can kidney beans, drained and rinsed

1 (28-ounce) can crushed tomatoes

1. Heat the oil in a large pot over medium heat. Add the onion and cook, stirring frequently, until soft, 4 to 5 minutes. Add the garlic and cook for 1 minute. Add the tomato paste and stir well.

2. Add the beef and cook, breaking it apart using a wooden spoon, until browned and cooked through, 8 to 10 minutes. Drain any excess fat and return the pot to the heat.

3. Add the chili powder, cumin, oregano, and paprika. Season with the salt and pepper to taste. Add the kidney beans and crushed tomatoes, stir to combine, and bring the chili to a boil. Cover the pot, reduce the heat to medium-low, and simmer for 20 to 25 minutes. Season with more salt and pepper, if desired. Spoon into bowls and serve.

LEFTOVER TIP: Store the chili in an airtight container in the refrigerator for up to 3 days.

PER SERVING: Calories: 215; Fat: 7g; Total Carbohydrates: 18g; Net Carbs: 11g; Fiber: 7g; Protein: 22g; Sodium: 272mg

BEEF LETTUCE WRAPS

Serves 4 · Prep time: 15 minutes / Cook time: 15 minutes
DAIRY-FREE, 30 MINUTES OR LESS

Lettuce wraps help reduce the amount of carbohydrates and total calories in a meal because lettuce is a substitute for bread. But if you need to increase the carbohydrates, use whole wheat tortillas instead of lettuce. Adjusting the amount of ground beef will help to raise or lower the protein content of this meal.

2 tablespoons creamy 100% all-natural peanut butter

2 tablespoons low-sodium soy sauce

½ teaspoon freshly squeezed lime juice

1 teaspoon sriracha

2 tablespoons water

1 tablespoon olive oil

2 scallions, green parts only, finely chopped

3 garlic cloves, minced

1 pound extra-lean ground beef

Sea salt

Freshly ground black pepper

1 cup canned sliced water chestnuts, drained

½ cup shredded carrots

12 large Butterhead lettuce leaves

3 tablespoons chopped peanuts

1. In a small bowl, mix the peanut butter, soy sauce, lime juice, sriracha, and water until mostly smooth. Set aside.

2. Heat the olive oil in a large nonstick skillet over medium-high heat. Add the scallions and garlic and sauté for 1 minute. Add the ground beef and cook, breaking it apart using a wooden spoon, until browned and cooked through, 8 to 10 minutes. Add salt and pepper to taste.

3. Add the peanut butter sauce, water chestnuts, and carrots and cook, stirring frequently, for 1 to 2 minutes.

4. Spoon the mixture into the lettuce leaves and garnish with the peanuts. Serve immediately.

> **SUBSTITUTION TIP:** These lettuce wraps can be made with extra-lean ground chicken, turkey, or pork (or a mixture) instead of ground beef.

PER SERVING: Calories: 326; Fat: 18g; Total Carbohydrates: 12g; Net Carbs: 9g; Fiber: 3g; Protein: 31g; Sodium: 451mg

PINEAPPLE, BELL PEPPER, AND BEEF BOWL

Serves 4 · Prep time: 10 minutes / Cook time: 35 minutes
DAIRY-FREE, GLUTEN-FREE

Simple meals make tracking macros easier, but simple does not mean your meals will be bland. Pineapple adds a punch of tangy flavor; its natural sugars help sweeten the meal and add a little zing.

1½ cups quinoa

1½ tablespoons olive oil, divided

1 pound extra-lean ground beef

½ teaspoon sea salt, plus more as needed

¼ teaspoon freshly ground black pepper, plus more as needed

2 green bell peppers, seeded and chopped

2 cups pineapple chunks

6 scallions, green parts only, thinly sliced

⅓ cup crushed unsalted cashews

1. Cook the quinoa according to the package instructions.

2. Heat 1 tablespoon of olive oil in a large nonstick skillet over medium-high heat. Add the ground beef, breaking it apart using a wooden spoon, and cook until browned and cooked through, 8 to 10 minutes. Add the salt and pepper and stir. Transfer to a plate and set aside.

3. In the same skillet, heat the remaining ½ tablespoon of olive oil. Add the bell peppers and sauté until tender, 4 to 6 minutes. Add the pineapple chunks and cook, stirring, for 1 minute.

4. Add the ground beef, scallions, and cashews to the skillet and cook, stirring, until blended, 1 to 2 minutes. Add salt and pepper to taste.

5. Divide the quinoa between 4 bowls. Top with the ground beef mixture and serve immediately.

> **SUBSTITUTION TIP:** If fresh pineapples are not available, use drained and rinsed canned pineapples instead.

PER SERVING: Calories: 553; Fat: 20g; Total Carbohydrates: 60g; Net Carbs: 52g; Fiber: 8g; Protein: 37g; Sodium: 319mg

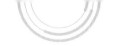

BEEF SPAGHETTI

Serves 4 · Prep time: 10 minutes / Cook time: 20 minutes
NUT-FREE

You can't go wrong with a classic spaghetti. If you're short on time, use a store-bought jarred pasta sauce and omit the crushed tomatoes, milk, and balsamic vinegar from this recipe. When selecting a sauce, be sure to choose one with lower sodium and no added sugars.

8 ounces whole-grain spaghetti

1 tablespoon olive oil, divided

1 pound extra-lean ground beef

Sea salt

Freshly ground black pepper

1 shallot, minced

3 garlic cloves, minced

1 cup sliced mushrooms

1½ cups crushed tomatoes

½ cup skim milk

2 teaspoons balsamic vinegar

1 tablespoon Italian seasoning

¼ cup grated reduced-fat Parmesan cheese

1. Cook the spaghetti according to the package instructions.

2. Heat ½ tablespoon of olive oil in a large nonstick skillet over medium-high heat. Add the ground beef, breaking it apart using a wooden spoon, and cook until browned and cooked through, 8 to 10 minutes. Drain any excess oil. Add salt and pepper and stir. Transfer to a plate and set aside.

3. In the same pan, heat the remaining ½ tablespoon of olive oil over medium-high heat. Add the shallot and sauté until soft, 1 to 2 minutes. Add the garlic and sauté for 1 minute. Add the mushrooms and sauté until soft, 2 to 3 minutes.

4. Add the crushed tomatoes, milk, balsamic vinegar, and Italian seasoning and mix well. Reduce the heat to low and cook until the sauce begins to thicken. Remove from the heat, add the ground beef, and mix well. Add salt and pepper to taste.

5. Divide the pasta between 4 bowls. Top with the beef mixture and top with the Parmesan cheese. Serve hot.

PER SERVING: Calories: 429; Fat: 11g; Total Carbohydrates: 49g; Net Carbs: 42g; Fiber: 7g; Protein: 36g; Sodium: 202mg

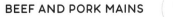

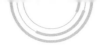

STUFFED ZUCCHINI BOATS

Makes 4 · Prep time: 15 minutes / Cook time: 1 hour
GLUTEN-FREE, NUT-FREE

Zucchini is a delicious low-calorie, low-carbohydrate vegetable. Spiralize them into noodles or, as in this recipe, use them as an edible shell to hold a tasty filling.

Nonstick cooking spray

2 medium zucchini, halved lengthwise

1 tablespoon olive oil

1 medium white onion, chopped

2 garlic cloves, minced

2 pounds extra-lean ground beef

1 yellow bell pepper, seeded and diced

1 large tomato, diced

1 teaspoon Italian seasoning

1 teaspoon ground cumin

1 teaspoon chili powder

Sea salt

Freshly ground black pepper

1 cup low-sodium marinara sauce

½ cup shredded reduced-fat mozzarella cheese

1. Preheat the oven to 400° F. Spray a baking dish with nonstick cooking spray.

2. Using a spoon, hollow out the center of each zucchini half to create 4 boats. Place them in the baking dish and set aside.

3. Heat the olive oil in a large nonstick skillet over medium-high heat. Add the onion and garlic and cook, stirring frequently, for 2 minutes. Add the ground beef, breaking it apart using a wooden spoon, and cook until browned and cooked through, 8 to 10 minutes. Drain any excess oil.

4. Add the bell pepper, tomato, Italian seasoning, cumin, and chili powder and stir to combine. Season with salt and pepper to taste. Cook for 2 minutes. Add the marinara sauce, lower the heat to medium-low, and simmer for 10 minutes. Remove the skillet from the heat, add the mozzarella cheese, and mix well.

5. Fill each zucchini boat with ¼ of the beef mixture and bake for 25 minutes, or until the zucchini are soft and cooked through. Serve immediately.

> **SUBSTITUTION TIP:** Don't have any mozzarella cheese on hand? Use the same amount of crumbled feta or shredded cheddar cheese.

PER SERVING: Calories: 432; Fat: 18g; Total Carbohydrates: 15g; Net Carbs: 11g; Fiber: 4g; Protein: 55g; Sodium: 277mg

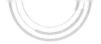

SPICY HONEY–MUSTARD PORK CHOPS

Serves 4 · Prep time: 10 minutes, plus 1 hour marinating /
Cook time: 10 minutes

DAIRY-FREE, GLUTEN-FREE, NUT-FREE

Marinades are a great way to impart flavor into meat, and they also keep meat tender and prevent it from drying out. These pork chops are delicious on their own or paired with a side salad or baked potato for a complete meal.

¼ cup Dijon mustard

1½ tablespoons honey

1 teaspoon freshly squeezed lemon juice

¼ teaspoon cayenne pepper

¼ teaspoon freshly ground black pepper

¼ teaspoon sea salt

4 (4-ounce) pork chops, 1 inch thick

2½ tablespoons olive oil, divided

2 garlic cloves, minced

3 cups sliced white button mushrooms

4 cups fresh baby spinach

1. Combine the mustard, honey, lemon juice, cayenne pepper, black pepper, and salt in a large zip-top plastic bag. Add the pork, remove as much air as possible, and seal. Carefully shake the bag a few times to coat the pork evenly with the marinade. Refrigerate for at least 1 hour.

2. Remove the pork chops from the plastic bag and discard the marinade. Heat 2 tablespoons of olive oil in a large nonstick skillet over medium heat. Add the pork chops and cook until they reach an internal temperature of 145° F, 4 to 6 minutes per side. Transfer the chops to a clean cutting board and let rest for 5 minutes before cutting them into slices.

3. In the same skillet, heat the remaining ½ tablespoon of olive oil. Add the garlic and sauté for 1 minute. Add the mushrooms and cook until soft, 2 to 3 minutes. Add the spinach and cook until it wilts, about 1 minute.

4. Divide the spinach between 4 plates and top with the pork chops.

> **LEFTOVER TIP:** Tightly wrap any leftover pork chops in aluminum foil or put them in an airtight container and refrigerate for up to 3 days.

PER SERVING: Calories: 305; Fat: 17g; Total Carbohydrates: 11g; Net Carbs: 9g; Fiber: 2g; Protein: 28g; Sodium: 370mg

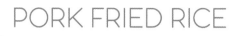

PORK FRIED RICE

Serves 4 · Prep time: 15 minutes / Cook time: 35 minutes
DAIRY-FREE, NUT-FREE

This recipe for fried rice packs in the carbohydrates, proteins, and healthy fats. Choose lean meats to keep the overall fat content down.

1 cup quick brown rice

1½ tablespoons olive oil

1 pound extra-lean
   ground pork

2 garlic cloves, minced

1 cup thinly sliced white
   button mushrooms

1 cup matchstick carrots

Sea salt

Freshly ground
   black pepper

2 tablespoons low-sodium
   soy sauce

4 scallions, green parts
   only, thinly sliced

1. Cook the rice according to the package instructions.

2. Heat a large nonstick skillet over medium-high heat until a drop of water sizzles on contact. Add 1 tablespoon of olive oil and use a small basting brush to coat the pan evenly. Add the ground pork, breaking it apart using a wooden spoon, and cook until browned and cooked through, 6 to 8 minutes. Transfer to a plate and set aside. Wipe out the skillet with paper towels and return it to the stovetop.

3. Heat the remaining ½ tablespoon of olive oil in the skillet over medium heat. Add the garlic and sauté for 1 minute. Add the mushrooms and carrots and cook, stirring occasionally, until the mushrooms are soft, 3 to 5 minutes. Season with salt and pepper to taste.

4. Return the pork to the skillet, add the rice and soy sauce, and cook, stirring constantly, until heated through, 1 to 2 minutes.

5. Divide the mixture between 4 bowls, garnish with the scallions, and serve.

SUBSTITUTION TIP: Try making this recipe with cooked quinoa or cooked farro instead of rice.

PER SERVING: Calories: 380; Fat: 11g; Total Carbohydrates: 42g; Net Carbs: 39g; Fiber: 3g; Protein: 29g; Sodium: 356mg

PORK AND ONION MEAT LOAF

Serves 6 • Prep time: 10 minutes / Cook time: 50 to 60 minutes
NUT-FREE

Here's another classic that you can absolutely eat while managing your macros. It's packed with protein, and you can raise or lower the amount of ground pork to meet your protein amount. Pair with roasted vegetables drizzled with olive oil to make this meal complete.

Nonstick cooking spray

2 pounds extra-lean ground pork

1 large egg, beaten

1 small white onion, chopped

½ cup skim milk

1 cup bread crumbs

½ teaspoon sea salt

¼ teaspoon freshly ground black pepper

⅓ cup barbecue sauce

1. Preheat the oven to 350°F. Lightly spray a baking dish with nonstick cooking spray.

2. In a large bowl, mix the ground pork, egg, onion, milk, bread crumbs, salt, and pepper.

3. Put the pork mixture into the baking dish.

4. Pour the barbecue sauce over the meat loaf, cover with aluminum foil, and bake for 50 to 60 minutes, or until cooked through.

> **SUBSTITUTION TIP:** If you don't like barbecue sauce, you can use ketchup or tomato sauce.

PER SERVING: Calories: 287; Fat: 8g; Total Carbohydrates: 19g; Net Carbs: 18g; Fiber: 1g; Protein: 36g; Sodium: 540mg

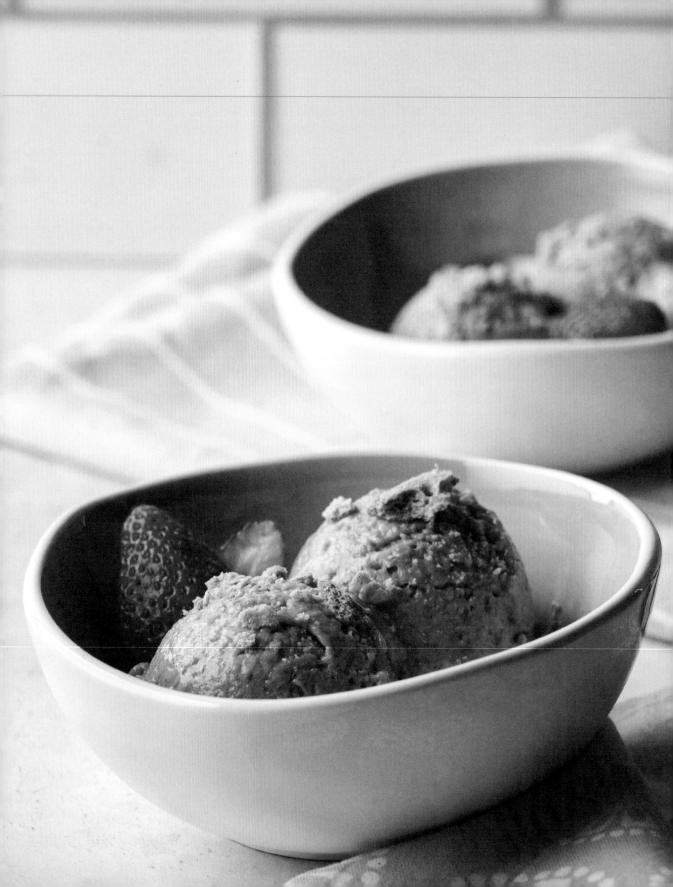

SWEETS

....

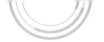

DARK CHOCOLATE–COVERED DATES

Makes 12 · Prep time: 10 minutes /
Cook time: 15 minutes, plus 30 minutes refrigeration

DAIRY-FREE, GLUTEN-FREE, VEGETARIAN

1 cup pitted dates

2 teaspoons
vanilla extract

12 pecan halves

¼ teaspoon sea salt

2½ ounces dark
chocolate

1. Line a baking sheet with parchment paper.

2. In a medium bowl, soak the dates in hot water
for 10 minutes.

3. In a food processor, combine the dates and
vanilla and puree until it reaches a jamlike consistency. You may need to stop and scrape down the
sides a few times.

4. Using your hands, form 12 marble-size balls
and place them on the prepared baking sheet.
Gently flatten the tops of the balls with your
fingers. Press 1 pecan half into each ball. Freeze
for 20 minutes.

5. In a small saucepan over low heat, combine the
salt and dark chocolate and stir until the chocolate is melted and smooth. Remove from the heat.
Using a small spoon, quickly pour a small amount
of dark chocolate over each pecan.

6. Return the baking sheet to the freezer for at least
10 minutes. Transfer the dates to an airtight container and refrigerate until ready to serve.

> **COOKING TIP:** Soaking dates in hot water for
> 10 minutes will make it easier to pulse with the
> vanilla in the food processor. Save 1 tablespoon of
> the soaking water, and if the mixture is too sticky to
> pulse, add a little more of the water.

PER SERVING (2 DATES): Calories: 99; Fat: 7g; Total Carbohydrates: 7g;
Net Carbs: 5g; Fiber: 2g; Protein: 1g; Sodium: 61mg

DARK CHOCOLATE–DRIZZLED STRAWBERRIES

Serves 4 · Prep time: 5 minutes /
Cook time: 5 minutes, plus 30 minutes refrigeration

NUT–FREE, VEGETARIAN

Strawberries are one of Mother Nature's candies. They can ramp up the sweetness of a dessert without greatly increasing your fat intake. It's also a satisfying dessert to serve to guests because they look fancy and—chocolate!

4 cups whole strawberries, rinsed and dried

2 ounces dark chocolate, broken into pieces

1. Line a baking sheet with parchment paper.

2. Put the strawberries on the prepared baking sheet.

3. In a microwave-safe bowl, melt the dark chocolate in 25-second intervals, stirring between each one, until smooth.

4. Using a spoon, quickly drizzle the chocolate over the strawberries. Refrigerate them for at least 30 minutes. Serve immediately or put them in an airtight container and refrigerate for up to 2 days.

> **SUBSTITUTION TIP:** If you are not a fan of strawberries, substitute 1½ cups fresh blueberries or raspberries. They are both fiber-rich fruits.

PER SERVING: Calories: 131; Fat: 6g; Total Carbohydrates: 18g; Net Carbs: 14g; Fiber: 4g; Protein: 2g; Sodium: 4mg

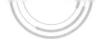

SALTED CARAMEL CASHEW BITES

Makes 7 cashew bites · Prep time: 15 minutes / Cook time: 20 minutes
DAIRY-FREE, GLUTEN-FREE, UNDER 40 MINUTES, VEGAN

Peanuts are actually legumes, making them higher in protein than other nuts. They also provide fiber and a variety of nutrients, including potassium, vitamin E, and magnesium.

1 cup pitted dates

2 teaspoons
  vanilla extract

1 tablespoon water

⅓ cup unsalted cashews

¼ cup raisins

⅛ cup peanuts

1. In a medium bowl, soak the dates in hot water for 10 minutes.

2. In a food processor, combine the dates, vanilla, and 1 tablespoon of water and process until it forms a paste. You may need to stop and scrape down the sides.

3. Add the cashews, raisins, and peanuts and continue to pulse until blended. Using your hands, form the mixture into 7 balls and put them on a plate. Refrigerate for at least 20 minutes before serving.

4. Store them in an airtight container in the refrigerator for up to 3 days.

> **COOKING TIP:** If you're looking to reduce the portion size to help meet your macronutrient ratio, roll the mixture into 14 smaller balls instead of 7.

PER SERVING (1 BITE): Calories: 116; Fat: 4g; Total Carbohydrates: 19g; Net Carbs: 17g; Fiber: 2g; Protein: 2g; Sodium: 3mg

SALTED PISTACHIO AND CRANBERRY CHOCOLATE COOKIES

Makes 12 cookies · Prep time: 10 minutes / Cook time: 20 minutes
30 MINUTES OR LESS, VEGETARIAN

If you're looking for a treat that delivers a perfect balance of sweet and salty, you will love these cookies. Pistachios pack in the protein, fiber, and antioxidants. If you'd like to lower the sugar and increase the healthy fat, omit the cranberries and use even more pistachios.

1¼ cups all-purpose flour

1 cup rolled oats

¼ cup packed
  brown sugar

¼ cup salted pistachios

¼ cup dried cranberries

2 tablespoons dark choc-
  olate chips

1 teaspoon baking powder

⅛ teaspoon sea salt

2 large eggs, beaten

¼ cup coconut oil, melted

1 teaspoon vanilla extract

1. Preheat the oven to 350° F. Line a baking sheet with parchment paper.

2. In a large bowl, mix the flour, oats, brown sugar, pistachios, cranberries, chocolate chips, baking powder, and salt.

3. In another bowl, mix the eggs, coconut oil, and vanilla. Pour the wet ingredients into the dry ingredients and mix until it forms a stiff dough. Using your hands, roll the mixture into 12 balls and put them on the prepared baking sheet. Using a spoon, flatten out the tops.

4. Bake for 18 to 20 minutes, or until lightly golden brown. Let cool on the baking sheet for 2 minutes before transferring them to a wire rack to cool completely. Store in an airtight container.

> **SUBSTITUTION TIP:** For a different flavor combination, try using raisins and walnuts instead of cranberries and pistachios.

PER SERVING (1 COOKIE): Calories: 174; Fat: 7g; Total Carbohydrates: 24g; Net Carbs: 22g; Fiber: 2g; Protein: 4g; Sodium: 49mg

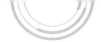

BLACK BEAN BROWNIE CUPS

Serves 8 · Prep time: 10 minutes / Cook time: 25 minutes
DAIRY-FREE, VEGAN

The not-so-secret ingredient in this recipe is black beans, which will help increase protein and fiber. The addition of the peanut butter and walnuts will increase the healthy fat content. And there's enough chocolate to make these irresistible.

Nonstick cooking spray

1 (15-ounce) can black beans, drained and rinsed

½ cup rolled oats

⅓ cup maple syrup

¼ cup olive oil

¼ cup creamy 100% all-natural peanut butter

2 tablespoons unsweetened cocoa powder

½ tablespoon vanilla extract

½ teaspoon baking powder

½ cup dark chocolate chips

¼ cup chopped walnuts

1. Preheat the oven to 350° F. Lightly spray a 12-cup muffin tin with nonstick cooking spray. Set aside.

2. In a food processor, combine the black beans, oats, maple syrup, olive oil, peanut butter, cocoa powder, vanilla, and baking powder and pulse until well combined.

3. Add the chocolate chips and pulse until combined. Transfer the brownie batter to a large bowl and fold in the walnuts. Divide the batter equally between the muffin cups.

4. Bake for 20 to 25 minutes, or until cooked. Let cool for 10 minutes before serving.

5. Refrigerate the brownies in an airtight container for up to 4 days.

> **COOKING TIP:** The brownie cups can be baked to your preferred texture—gooey brownies will bake for about 20 minutes, while firmer brownies will bake closer to 25 minutes.

PER SERVING: Calories: 303; Fat: 18g; Total Carbohydrates: 29g; Net Carbs: 23g; Fiber: 6g; Protein: 8g; Sodium: 6mg

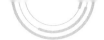

FRUIT SKEWERS WITH CHIA YOGURT DIP

Serves 4 · Prep time: 5 minutes / Cook time: 5 minutes
30 MINUTES OR LESS, VEGETARIAN

Here's a way to dress up fruit—and serve it with a dip that won't pack in any added sugar but will add some protein. Chia seeds increase the nutritional value of the dip by adding fiber.

2 bananas, cut into
   1-inch slices
6 large strawberries,
   stemmed and halved
2 kiwis, peeled and cut
   into quarters
½ cup fresh blueberries
½ cup nonfat plain
   Greek yogurt
1 tablespoon maple syrup
½ tablespoon chia seeds
2 tablespoons unsweet-
   ened cocoa powder
½ teaspoon vanilla extract
½ ounce 70% dark
   chocolate

1. Thread the bananas, strawberries, kiwis, and blueberries onto 4 skewers. Set aside.

2. In a small bowl, mix the yogurt, maple syrup, chia seeds, cocoa powder, and vanilla. Set aside.

3. In a microwave-safe bowl, melt the dark chocolate in 25-second intervals, stirring between each one, until melted.

4. Add the chocolate to the yogurt mixture and quickly stir until combined.

5. Serve immediately with the chocolate and yogurt sauce on the side.

COOKING TIP: There are a few ways to increase the sweetness of this dip: increase the maple syrup to 2 teaspoons; use 50% dark chocolate instead of 70%; or use ½ reduced-sugar vanilla Greek yogurt and ½ plain Green yogurt. Remember, any modifications will change the nutritional value.

PER SERVING: Calories: 139; Fat: 3g; Total Carbohydrates: 27g; Net Carbs: 23g; Fiber: 4g; Protein: 5g; Sodium: 13mg

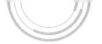

CINNAMON-OAT BAKED PEAR

Serves 6 · Prep time: 5 minutes / Cook time: 30 minutes

DAIRY-FREE, VEGAN

Pears are a great fall fruit that can be consumed as is or dressed up with spices, like the cinnamon in this recipe. If you're looking to limit your sugar intake, omit or reduce the amount of raisins. If you're looking to increase the fat content, add more walnuts. To increase the protein content, pair the pear (pun intended) with nonfat plain Greek yogurt.

2 tablespoons rolled oats

2 tablespoons
   crushed walnuts

1 tablespoon raisins

1 tablespoon maple syrup

1 teaspoon vanilla extract

¼ teaspoon ground cin-
   namon, plus more for
   sprinkling (optional)

3 large pears, halved
   and cored

1. Preheat the oven to 350° F. Line a baking sheet with parchment paper.

2. In a small bowl, mix the oats, walnuts, raisins, maple syrup, vanilla, and cinnamon. Set aside.

3. Cut a small sliver off the back of each pear to allow pears to sit flat on the prepared baking sheet. Spoon the oat mixture into the center of each pear half and sprinkle with more cinnamon, if using.

4. Bake for 25 to 30 minutes, or until soft and lightly browned.

5. Put the pears on plates, making sure to top them with any remaining mixture. Serve immediately.

> **SUBSTITUTION TIP:** Not a fan of pears? Try using another favorite fall fruit, like apples. Bake them for about 30 to 40 minutes, or until tender.

PER SERVING: Calories: 107; Fat: 1g; Total Carbohydrates: 24g; Net Carbs: 20g; Fiber: 4g; Protein: 1g; Sodium: 2mg

STRAWBERRY SHORTCAKE NICE CREAM

Serves 2 · Prep time: 5 minutes / Cook time: 10 minutes
NUT-FREE, 30 MINUTES OR LESS, VEGETARIAN

Nice cream is a low-fat frozen dessert that really satisfies on those days when you're craving something sweet. Frozen bananas deliver the same consistency as soft serve or ice cream, making this a fun treat.

2 large frozen bananas,
**   cut into slices**
2 tablespoons 1% milk
1½ cups stemmed and
**   halved strawberries**
6 graham crackers

1. In a food processor, combine the bananas and milk and pulse until smooth and creamy. If you like a thicker consistency, omit the milk. Add the strawberries and 4 of the graham crackers and continue to pulse until well combined.

2. Divide the mixture between 2 bowls. Break the remaining graham crackers into small pieces, sprinkle over the top, and serve.

> **LEFTOVER TIP:** The nice cream can be stored in an airtight container and frozen. After 4 hours in the freezer, it will have the consistency of traditional, harder ice cream.
>
> **PREP TIP:** You can also use frozen strawberries for a consistency even closer to ice cream.

PER SERVING: Calories: 257; Fat: 4g; Total Carbohydrates: 57g; Net Carbs: 50g; Fiber: 7g; Protein: 4g; Sodium: 105mg

GOAT CHEESE AND TOMATO
BREAKFAST WRAP • PAGE 51

MEASUREMENT CONVERSIONS

Volume Equivalents (Liquid)

US STANDARD	US STANDARD (OUNCES)	METRIC (APPROX.)
2 tablespoons	1 fl. oz.	30 mL
¼ cup	2 fl. oz.	60 mL
½ cup	4 fl. oz.	120 mL
1 cup	8 fl. oz.	240 mL
1½ cups	12 fl. oz.	355 mL
2 cups or 1 pint	16 fl. oz.	475 mL
4 cups or 1 quart	32 fl. oz.	1 L
1 gallon	128 fl. oz.	4 L

Oven Temperatures

FAHRENHEIT (F)	CELSIUS (C) (APPROX.)
250°	120°
300°	150°
325°	165°
350°	180°
375°	190°
400°	200°
425°	220°
450°	230°

Volume Equivalents (Dry)

US STANDARD	METRIC (APPROX.)
⅛ teaspoon	0.5 mL
¼ teaspoon	1 mL
½ teaspoon	2 mL
¾ teaspoon	4 mL
1 teaspoon	5 mL
1 tablespoon	15 mL
¼ cup	59 mL
¾ cup	79 mL
½ cup	118 mL
⅔ cup	156 mL
¾ cup	177 mL
1 cup	235 mL
2 cups or 1 pint	475 mL
3 cups	700 mL
4 cups or 1 quart	1 L

Weight Equivalents

US STANDARD	METRIC (APPROX.)
½ ounce	15 g
1 ounce	30 g
2 ounces	60 g
4 ounces	115 g
8 ounces	225 g
12 ounces	340 g
16 ounces or 1 pound	455 g

RESOURCES

GENERAL NUTRITION

With access to infinite dietary information at our fingertips, it's important to obtain information from reputable sources. These resources will provide you with sound nutritional information and the current food and nutrition guidelines for the United States and Canada.

→ Academy of Nutrition and Dietetics: Complete Food and Nutrition Guide: EatRight.org

→ Canada's Food Guide: Food-Guide.Canada.ca/en

→ Dietary Guidelines for Americans: Health.gov/our-work/food-nutritio n/2015-2020-dietary-guidelines

ACTIVITY GUIDELINES

Nutrition and physical activity are both important components of a healthy life-style. The resources below are guidelines used in the United States and Canada to help optimize the health benefits associated with physical activity.

→ Physical Activity Guidelines for Americans: Health.gov/our-work /physical-activity/current-guidelines

→ Canadian 24-Hour Movement Guidelines: CSEPGuidelines.ca

WEBSITES & APPS

For easy access to food information, nutrient profiles, macro tracking, and calculating your estimated energy needs, websites and apps can be very useful. The following resources are easy to navigate and can help provide dietary information.

→ Best Food Facts: BestFoodFacts.org

→ National Institute of Diabetes and Digestive Kidney Disease: Body Weight Planner: NIDDK.NIH.gov/bwp

→ USDA FoodData Central: FDC.nal.usda.gov

→ MyFitnessPal: MyFitnessPal.com

→ Macros Calorie Counter: apps.apple.com/ca/app /macros-calorie-counter/id1216666985

→ MyPlate Calorie Counter: apps.apple.com/ca/app /myplate-calorie-counter/id502317923

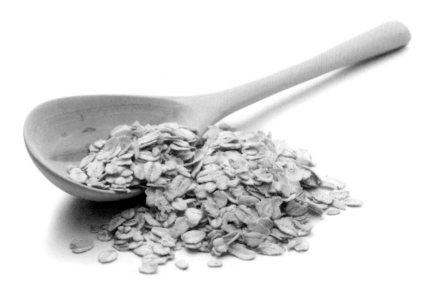

REFERENCES

Canadian Society for Exercise Physiology. "Canadian Physical Activity Guidelines for Adults (18–64 years)." Accessed September 10, 2020. CSEPGuidelines.ca /adults-18-64.

Duyff, Roberta L. *Academy of Nutrition and Dietetics: Complete Food and Nutrition Guide,* 5th Edition. New York: Houghton Mifflin Harcourt Publishing Company, 2017.

Gardner C. D., J. F. Trepanowski, L. C. Del Gobbo, et al. "Effect of Low-Fat vs Low-Carbohydrate Diet on 12-Month Weight Loss in Overweight Adults and the Association With Genotype Pattern or Insulin Secretion: The DIETFITS Randomized Clinical Trial." *JAMA* 319, no. 7 (2018): 667–679, doi:10.1001 /jama.2018.0245.

Gottschlich, Michele M, Mark H. DeLegge, Todd Mattox, Charles Mueller, Patricia Washington, and P. Guenter. "Calculation Methods to Determine Energy Expenditure for Healthy Individuals" in *The A.S.P.E.N. NUTRITION SUPPORT CORE CURRICULUM: A CASE-BASED APPROACH—THE ADULT PATIENT.* American Society for Parenteral and Enteral Nutrition: USA, 25.

Heart and Stroke Canada. "Reduce Sugar." Accessed September 29, 2020. HeartandStroke.CA/get-healthy/healthy-eating/reduce-sugar.

Kelly, Mark. "Resting Metabolic Rate: Best Ways to Measure It and Raise It, Too." American Council on Exercise. Accessed September 10, 2020. ACEFitness.org /certifiednewsarticle/2882/resting-metabolic-rate-best-ways-to-measure-it-and -raise-it-too.

Office of Disease Prevention, US Department of Health. *Dietary Guidelines for Americans 2015–2020,* 8th Edition. "Daily Nutrition Goals for Age-Sex Groups Based on Dietary Reference Intakes and Dietary Guideline Recommendations." Accessed September 4, 2020. Health.gov/our-work/food-nutrition/2015-2020 -dietary-guidelines/guidelines/appendix-7.

Sacks, F. M., G. A. Bray, V. J. Carey, S. R. Smith, D. H. Ryan, S. D. Anton, K. McManus, C. M. Champagne, L. M. Bishop, N. Laranjo, M. S. Leboff, J. C. Rood, L. de Jonge, F. L. Greenway, C. M. Loria, E. Obarzanek, and D. A. Williamson. "Comparison of Weight-Loss Diets with Different Compositions of Fat, Protein, and Carbohydrates." *The New England Journal of Medicine*, 360, no/ 9 (2009): 859–873, doi: 10.1056/NEJMoa0804748.

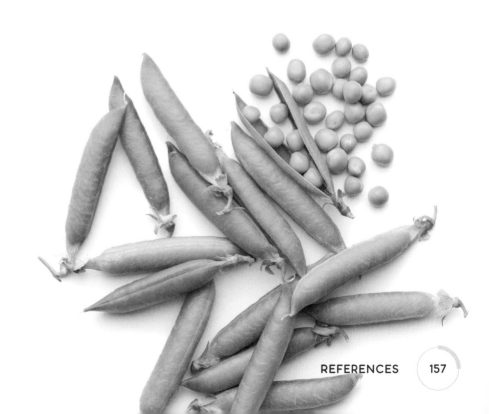

INDEX

ABOUT THE AUTHOR

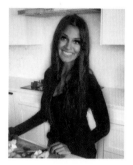

DEVIKA SHARMA is a registered dietitian and founder of One More Bite Nutrition, a nutrition consulting company specializing in portion-control methods for weight management. With close to a decade of work experience, she has been working with people to help them understand the importance of balanced eating. This has made her an inspiring health coach in the industry as she continues to support sustainable weight goals while enjoying a variety of foods that accommodate different lifestyles. She is also the coauthor of *The Healthy Indian*, a cookbook designed to help readers enjoy classic Indian meals while meeting nutrition goals. Devika believes that you *can* have your cake and eat it, too, when managing weight—*finally*! Devika can be found on Instagram (@nutritionbydevika), Facebook (@nutritionbydevika), or at www.OneMoreBite.ca.

ACKNOWLEDGMENTS

I would like to express my sincere gratitude to all the people who have supported me through this publication process. I am especially grateful to Callisto Media for giving me the opportunity to write this book. Adrian Potter and Kelly Koester, I couldn't have done this without you!

I would also like to thank my family, Rishi and Jehan Sharma, Suresh Sharma, and Nittan and Vinita Sood, for the support and taste-testing all my recipes. A special thanks to my mom, Amita Sharma, who I know would be very proud of this accomplishment if she were here today.